John Eden is the Associate Professor in Reproduction at the University of New South Wales and the Director of the Sydney Menopause Centre, the Natural Therapies Unit and the Barbara Gross Research Unit, all located at the Royal Hospital for Women in Sydney. He was one of the first certified reproductive endocrinologists in Australia and is the recipient of a number of awards and prizes, including the President's Prize from the Royal Society of Medicine in London for his research into ovarian growth factors, the Fotheringham Fellowship from the Royal Australian and New Zealand College of Obstetricians and Gynaecologists, and the CIBA Menopause Award from the Australasian Menopause Society. He was also appointed to the Executive Council of the Australasian Menopause Society for many years and was a member of the Australian Medical Association's Committee on Complementary Medicines. Dr Eden was a member of the Australian government committee that examined complementary medicines (Expert Committee on Complementary Medicines in the Health System), following the Pan Pharmaceutical investigation of 2003.

Dr Eden's ongoing research includes the causes of polycystic ovary syndrome, the impact of diet on the reproductive system, hormones and their effect on breast cancer, menopausal imbalances and herbal medicines. He has published many articles in major scientific journals relating to women's hormones, and also serves as a referee for a number of scientific journals and organisations, vetting the articles of other medical journalists and specialists. Because of his expertise in these medical fields, Dr Eden regularly delivers talks to medical organisations, national and international scientific conferences and women's groups, and is often interviewed on radio and television.

Note on the availability of contraceptive pills

Not all the contraceptive pills listed in this book are available in the United States, in particular, Diane-35 is not available. I therefore recommend that patients ask their doctors for Yasmin. Although Yasmin does not contain CPA (cytoperone acetate), it has been shown to give good results for women with PCO and PCOS and I do recommend it to my own patients.

Note on measurements

Where applicable, I have included measurement conversions to give international readers the imperial and US equivalents to the SI metric measurements used in studies and tables in this book. In general the SI metric units are listed first, with the US equivalents enclosed in brackets immediately after. However, as not all pathologists use the same units, it is always advisable to discuss your test results with your own doctor.

Polycystic Ovary Syndrome

A woman's guide to identifying and managing PCOS

Dr John Eden

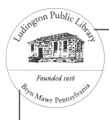

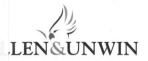

ALLEN&UNWIN

The information in this book is intended as a guide only, and should not substitute medical advice or care. Always consult your doctor in the first instance.

First published in Australia in 2005

Allen & Unwin
83 Alexander Street
Crows Nest NSW 2065
Australia
Phone: (61 2) 8425 0100
Fax: (61 2) 9906 2218
Email: info@allenandunwin.com
Web: www.allenandunwin.com

National Library of Australia
Cataloguing-in-Publication entry:

Eden, John A.
Polycystic ovary syndrome : a woman's guide to identifying and managing PCOS

Bibliography.
Includes index.
ISBN 1 74114 527 9.

1. Polycystic ovary syndrome – Popular works. 2. Ovaries – Diseases – Popular works. I. Title.

618.11

Index by Russell Brooks
Typeset in 13/16 pt Granjon by Midland Typesetters, Maryborough
Printed by CMO Image Printing Enterprise, Singapore
10 9 8 7 6 5 4 3 2

Contents

Figures and tables   viii

Preface   xi

1   Making sense of alphabet soup: Polycystic ovaries
and polycystic ovary syndrome explained   1
     What is a polycystic ovary?   1
     What is polycystic ovary syndrome?   4
     How does the menstrual cycle work?   6
     Summary   15
     Frequently asked questions   17

2   Looking for signs: PCO and PCOS diagnosed   19
     How can doctors see an ovary?   20
     Do I have polycystic ovaries?   21
     Do I have polycystic ovary syndrome?   22
     Summary   29
     Frequently asked questions   30

3 Searching for answers: Causes of polycystic ovary
   syndrome   32
   Are my genes to blame?   32
   Do I have too many male hormones?   37
   Is it my brain hormones?   38
   Did it happen before I was born?   39
   Was it something I ate?   39
   Does insulin resistance affect PCOS?   43
   Summary   44
   Frequently asked questions   44

4 Scratching below the surface: Skin and hair symptoms   46
   Why does hair grow or not grow?   46
   Why is my face breaking out all the time?   50
   Do hormones affect the skin and hair?   53
   Which hormonal tests should I have?   55
   How do you treat hair and skin problems?   57
   Summary   69
   Frequently asked questions   70

5 Counting the days: Menstrual irregularities   72
   Why do many women with PCOS have a menstrual
   problem?   73
   What else causes menstrual irregularities?   80
   What can I do to control menstrual problems?   101
   Summary   108
   Frequently asked questions   109

6 Producing results: Fertility issues   110
   Am I infertile?   111
   Do I need contraception?   112
   But what if I want to have a baby?   122
   Do PCO and PCOS affect pregnancy outcomes?   142
   Summary   144
   Frequently asked questions   145

7 Taking the sugar: The diet and insulin story   148
   What is insulin resistance?   149
   How do I control and prevent insulin resistance?   156
   What surgical procedures are available for weight loss?   170
   Summary   172
   Frequently asked questions   172

8 Protecting yourself: Potential long-term health issues   174
   What is my risk of osteoporosis?   175
   What is my risk of cancer?   176
   What is my risk of heart and blood vessel disease, and
   diabetes?   177
   Summary   178
   Frequently asked questions   178

9 Tapping into the future: Potential new treatments   180
   What will research unveil?   181
   What new medical breakthroughs are likely?   183
   What is your final summary?   183

Glossary and abbreviations   186
References and further reading   193
Useful websites   201
Index   206

Figures and tables

Figures

1.1	A normal ovary and a polycystic ovary	2
1.2	The location of the endocrine glands	8
1.3	The hypothalamic-pituary-ovarian axis	13
1.4	Control of follicular growth in the ovary	14
3.1	Causes of PCO	43
4.1	Hair follicle	47
4.2	The effect of testosterone on skin	55
4.3	The contraceptive Pill and CPA	64
5.1	The effect of diet and insulin on free testosterone	74
5.2	The effect of weight change on testosterone and menstruation	75
5.3	Pelvic causes of abnormal bleeding	96
5.4	Endometriosis	99
5.5	Hysterectomy	108
6.1	Basal body temperature chart (BBTc)	124
7.1	The impact of IR and excessively raised insulin levels	151
7.2	Insulin resistance	156

7.3   Insulin and LH both stimulate the ovary to
       make testosterone   165

Tables

1.1   Factors influencing levels of SHBG and free
       testosterone   10
1.2   The main functions of the sex hormones   12
2.1   Basic blood tests for menstrual irregularities   24
2.2   Quick guide to what blood tests for PCOS might
       reveal   25
2.3   Beth's blood test results   27
3.1   Results of ultrasound scanning for PCO   35
3.2   Sheep clover disease and human PCOS   41
4.1   Average results for women with excess body hair   50
4.2   The Marynick acne scoring system   51
4.3   Average blood results   52
4.4   The effect of Androcur treatment on average (range)
       acne scores   53
4.5   The effects of oestrogen and testosterone on skin   54
5.1   Menstrual regularity of women in the 'thousand
       cases of PCOS' research   76
5.2   Clinical and hormonal data (expressed as averages)
       from the 'thousand cases of PCOS' research   77
5.3   Jessie's blood test results   82
5.4   Examples of Synacthen test results   94
6.1   Infertility causes of 144 women with PCOS   112
6.2   Nathalie's blood test results   129
6.3   Katie's blood test results   132
6.4   Types of FSH therapy   135
6.5   Danielle's blood test results   139
6.6   Laparoscopic surgery to induce ovulation   142
7.1   Glucose tolerance test 1 results   153
7.2   Glucose tolerance test 2 results   153

7.3	Glucose tolerance test 3 results	154
7.4	Glucose tolerance test 4 results	154
7.5	Glucose tolerance test 5 results	155
7.6	Examples of GI-rated foods	163
7.7	Kathy's baseline blood test results	167
7.8	Jenny's initial hormone results	169
7.9	Jenny's GTT results	169

Preface

Up until the last few decades, medicine was taught much like an apprenticeship. The student learnt from a professor and the word of the professor was not to be questioned. Then along came evidence-based medicine—a new way of thinking. The evidence is gathered not from the professor's viewpoint, but rather from the results of:

- randomised controlled trials (RCTs), where half the participants receive the active treatment and the other half are given a dummy treatment;
- population studies, where a group of people who suffer from a condition is compared with a similar group of people (i.e. same age and gender) who do not suffer from the condition in order to collect statistical data on such things as side-effects;
- case reports of patients who suffer from an illness;
- laboratory and animal studies; and
- the opinions of various experts.

The best evidence is obtained from RCTs, followed by population studies and then case studies. Evidence-based medicine constantly questions the existing view of diagnosis and treatment. There are still many who cling to the prevailing doctrines, but evidence-based research cuts through personal viewpoints and biases. Insight and experience are valuable tools for generating ideas, but evidence-based research is able to prove these ideas.

Someone once said that there are three types of knowledge: objective (you can measure something—e.g. evidence-based medicine); intellectual (e.g. maths—you can do the sums, but can't 'touch it'); and finally experiential (based on emotions and experience). All of these are important. For example, the medical evidence suggests that the contraceptive Pill is useful for a problem such as heavy irregular periods. However, a particular woman's experience, religious beliefs or culture might make the Pill unacceptable for her. Thus health science meets the art of healing.

Reproductive endocrinology, or the study of women's hormonal patterns, has benefited enormously from evidence-based medicine. It is a relatively new specialty, but the problems that can occur in this area of health—infertility, erratic menopausal symptoms and menstrual irregularities—have been around forever. This is also one area of medicine where far too many urban and medical myths have evolved, and these need to be addressed. This is especially so for polycystic ovary syndrome (PCOS). As a specialist in women's hormones, it seems to me that nearly every person has an opinion about PCOS, and much of what I am told each day is simply not true. It is my hope that this book will dispel many of these misleading myths. It is also important to deal with a woman's fears.

Population studies using ultrasound scans have shown that up to one in four women could be diagnosed as having polycystic ovaries (PCO). This fact, together with the name itself—'polycystic ovaries'—sounds alarming. What is more alarming, though, is the amount of women who come to me totally misinformed about this condition. After being told their ovaries have 'cysts' on them, they are fearful because they've heard they will need extensive surgery to fix this. Some women believe they are infertile, when most are not. Some are told that PCOS will make them obese, and if their ovaries are removed, they will find it easier to lose the excess weight. Or they read on websites that they will develop diabetes or die prematurely of heart disease. These and other mostly inaccurate pronouncements by friends, family and the media are not helpful. Even some good doctors may unintentionally add to the confusion around PCOS.

Myth: Few women have polycystic ovaries.
Fact: About one in four women of reproductive age have PCO.

While specialist doctors like myself don't have all the facts yet about this common condition, we have learnt an awful lot during the past twenty years, mostly through evidence-based medicine. This new information is producing a lot of hope and comfort, rather than despair and fear. Now I would like to share with you what we do know about this syndrome and what we are learning and hope to be able to offer in the future so that you will be able to sort your way through the minefield of myths out there.

I would very much like to thank the thousands of women who have come to see me as patients over the years. It is because of them that I have been able to gather this wealth of information, and in turn it has helped many others who suffer from the effects of this syndrome. I would also like to thank my research staff and students who have helped me with the various research projects described in this book. Many people encouraged me to write this book. I would like to thank all the staff at the Royal Hospital for Women who have supported me in my work and throughout the writing process. I would also like to thank my wife, Barbara, and my children for putting up with the many intrusions it has made into our family life.

I hope you find the information of great value.

John Eden

1
Making sense of alphabet soup:
Polycystic ovaries and polycystic ovary syndrome explained

Unfortunately, we doctors often give diseases names which sound very threatening and then, to make matters even worse, we turn them into confusing acronyms. The term 'polycystic ovary', or PCO, is a good example of this. For good measure, let's add the word 'syndrome' and it becomes polycystic ovary syndrome, or PCOS. It sounds painful—as if the ovary is constantly full of large, painful cysts—and even hints at the threat of radical surgery. However, neither of these scenarios is true.

What is a polycystic ovary?

The possibility that a woman may have polycystic ovaries is one of the most common reasons for a GP to refer someone to my clinical practice. Many of these women arrive confused and often very frightened. They have usually gone to their GP because their periods are irregular or because they have concerns about an excessive amount of body hair (hirsutism) and/or acne (see Chapters 4 and 5 for a more detailed discussion of these symptoms). Then they are confronted with a medical term they may not have heard about before and they dread a prognosis, sometimes linking the condition with cancer. Fortunately, it usually takes just a little accurate information to allay their fears.

The ovary is a dynamic organ, changing its shape and appearance according to its hormonal environment. We can look at a woman's ovaries through two common procedures: ultrasound scanning; and a laparoscopy, a keyhole surgical technique where a telescope is inserted into the abdominal cavity via a small cut in the navel (under a full anaesthetic). In practice, ultrasound is by far the most common way of finding polycystic ovaries. A five-year-old girl's ovaries are inactive and small, with a volume of only 1–2 millilitres or 0.03–0.07 fluid ounces (a teaspoon holds 5 millilitres/0.2 fluid ounces). During a woman's reproductive years, each of her ovaries has a volume of around 4–6 millilitres (0.13–0.2 fluid ounces) and they have a convoluted, folded surface which looks a bit like the surface of a walnut (see Figure 1).

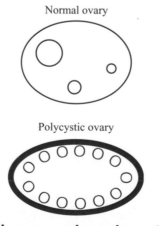

Normal ovary

Polycystic ovary

Figure 1.1 A normal ovary and a polycystic ovary

Ovulating ovaries contain fluid-filled structures called follicles, which may vary in size from 1–30 millimetres (0.04–1.18 inches), depending on the phase of the menstrual cycle. Each of these follicles contains a microscopic egg, and there are usually between two and five of them scattered throughout the ovaries. In contrast, the polycystic ovary typically has more than twelve small follicles, each around 2–9 millimetres (0.08–0.35 inches) in diameter, which are usually arranged in a 'pearl-necklace' pattern. A polycystic ovary is also usually larger than normal, with a volume of more than 10 millilitres (0.34 fluid ounces) and has a smooth thick surface, or capsule. Often this capsule is covered in tiny blood vessels.

The name 'polycystic ovary' is an unfortunate one, as the ovary is actually not full of cysts. In medical terminology, the term 'cyst' normally refers to a fluid-filled structure more than 30 millimetres (1.18 inches) in diameter. So, strictly speaking, polycystic ovaries do not have cysts; it is the particular follicular pattern and number of follicles that defines the condition.

Myth: Polycystic ovaries are full of cysts.
Fact: The term PCO refers to a pattern of twelve or more small (2–6 millimetre/0.08–0.24 inch) follicles arranged around the periphery of the ovary in a pearl-necklace pattern. They are not technically 'cysts', and do not need to be removed surgically.

The follicles of polycystic ovaries behave differently, in the reproductive sense, to normal follicles. If you have polycystic ovaries, you certainly do not need surgery to remove the follicles, and you are also not at increased risk of cancer of the ovaries. We will go into more detail about this later.

> **Myth:** Women with polycystic ovaries have cysts which need to be removed through surgery.
> **Fact:** The so-called 'cysts' are actually small follicles, each containing an egg. There is no need for surgery to remove the follicles from an ovary: they are a normal part of an ovulating ovary.

What is polycystic ovary syndrome?

It is very important to distinguish between polycystic ovaries (PCO) and polycystic ovary syndrome (PCOS). Having PCO does not necessarily mean you have PCOS. A syndrome is usually defined as a pattern of symptoms belonging to a particular disease. Medical studies using ultrasound have found that around one in four women has polycystic ovaries, but most of them have none or few of the other symptoms associated with polycystic ovary syndrome. The main features of PCOS are male hormone excess and polycystic ovaries. Some of the problems that women with PCOS may have include:

- excess hair on the body (hirsutism);
- acne and other skin problems;
- scalp hair loss;
- irregular or missing periods;
- heavy periods;
- fertility problems;
- insulin resistance;
- weight issues.

Some of these symptoms, such as excess body hair, will depend on the person's genetic makeup. For example, Asiatic people are not very hairy, so Chinese women with PCOS rarely suffer from this symptom, whereas people from the Mediterranean do have much more body hair, so excess body hair is likely to be a sign. It is the symptoms, not necessarily the realisation that they may have polycystic ovaries, that cause women to seek medical help. As discussed, polycystic ovaries are not painful and most women do not know they have them until a symptom of the syndrome becomes a concern. During the process of treating the symptom, they discover they have PCO or PCOS.

Until 2003, there was a worldwide consensus that PCOS was diagnosed only when a woman had fewer than six menstrual cycles per year and the visual telltale sign on the ovary (twelve or more small follicles in a 'necklace' pattern) could be seen on an ultrasound. In the United States, where ultrasound is not usually performed, the diagnosis was made when an excess of the male hormone (androgen) was discovered either through the observation of excessive hair growth or via raised male hormones in a blood test, as well as fewer than six periods per year (see Chapter 2 for more details on diagnosis). While polycystic ovaries are common—with one in four women having them—only about 7 per cent of women in the reproductive age group will have PCOS—that is, PCO and fewer than six periods per year.

That all changed in 2003. A meeting of international experts resulted in a revision of the definitions. The paper they published (see Rotterdam ESHRE/ASRM-Sponsored Consensus PCOS Workshop Group, 2004) stated that: 'PCOS is a syndrome of ovarian dysfunction. Its cardinal features are hyperandrogenism and polycystic morphology.' This means that PCOS is characterised by the ovaries not working properly, an excess of male hormones (as measured on a blood test or implied by the presence of excess body hair) and a polycystic appearance of the ovaries.

It is worth noting at this point that any menstrual irregularity could be a symptom of another hormone problem such as early menopause, and excess androgen could also be caused by the adrenal gland over-producing the male hormones, rather than by PCOS. Hormonal-related symptoms therefore have to be carefully scrutinised before a diagnosis of PCOS is made to eliminate all other possible causes. We will discuss all these symptoms in greater detail later, but in order to understand PCO and PCOS it is important to go back to the basics—to understand how the female reproductive system actually works.

Myth: All women with PCO have PCOS.
Fact: PCOS is diagnosed only when two of the following three symptoms are present and other causes are excluded:
- irregular periods (usually fewer than six periods per year);
- blood tests or symptoms suggesting male hormone excess;
- polycystic ovaries.

How does the menstrual cycle work?

Menstruation is an incredibly complex process. The first period, called the *menarche*, usually occurs around the age of twelve years, but most young women notice some breast development around the age of ten, and soon after that hair starts to grow in the armpits and groin. Just before menarche, girls experience a growth spurt, initiated by *human growth hormone* (HGH), a hormone produced by the pituitary gland. Generally, growth will start to slow at the onset of the first period as a rise in levels of *oestrogen* (another female hormone) fuses the growth plates (located at the ends of the long bones in the arms and legs), turning them into bone, thus preventing further growth.

A menstrual cycle occurs roughly in a monthly pattern (typically a 28-day cycle, but usually anywhere between 21 and 35 days). In the first half of the cycle, oestrogen levels rise, causing the *endometrium* (the lining of the uterus) to thicken. *Ovulation* occurs in the middle of the cycle (about day 14), when oestrogen levels peak, and after this large amounts of a second female hormone, *progesterone*, are produced from the emptied follicle, now called the *corpus luteum*. Progesterone causes the endometrium to stop thickening and to become receptive to a possible embryo. Progesterone also prevents menstruation if a woman becomes pregnant, and it is associated with premenstrual fluid retention and often some bowel bloating and period pain. About a week before a period is due, progesterone levels start to drop if pregnancy has not occurred. Once a period has started, oestrogen begins to rise again, starting a new cycle.

As you can see, hormones are incredibly important in the menstrual process and for many other body functions.

What are hormones?

Our body is made up of billions and billions of cells, and these cells need to communicate with each other so that everything functions in unison. The body is a bit like an orchestra, with each instrument representing an individual cell. The orchestra needs to follow the conductor to produce a beautiful piece of music. If the instruments are not coordinated, then a terrible noise results. Likewise, if the cells in our bodies are not properly coordinated, we become sick.

The body uses two main communication systems in order to keep in sync: the nervous system and hormones. The nervous system is hard-wired into the body and permits rapid commands and responses. For example, if you step onto something sharp, pain sensors in the skin of your foot rapidly let your brain know something is wrong. The brain in turn rapidly responds by activating the appropriate leg muscles to withdraw your foot—and this all happens in a split second. Hormones, on the other hand, are chemical messengers that travel from one part of the body to another to either stimulate or inhibit an 'everyday' action in the body. The effects of hormones appear more slowly and last for longer than nervous stimuli, and they are usually apparent in tissues quite remote from the gland where they originated.

Hormones are produced in the *endocrine glands*—pineal, pituitary, thyroid, parathyroid, adrenal, pancreas and ovaries or testes (see Figure 1.2). Each gland is responsible for the production of specific hormones that control important and widely different processes such as nutrition, growth and reproduction.

The principal endocrine gland is the *pituitary*, located behind the nose at the bottom of the brain. The pituitary is responsible for controlling all the other major glands in the body, releasing a variety of hormones to control the ovaries (and testicles), the thyroid glands, the adrenals and so on. For example, the pituitary gland releases the *follicle stimulating hormone* (FSH), which stimulates the small follicles to grow in size—hence its name. FSH also stimulates the ovary to produce and release oestrogen. Oestrogen, like progesterone and androgens, is a sex hormone. Sex hormones, as the name suggests, govern our reproductive system.

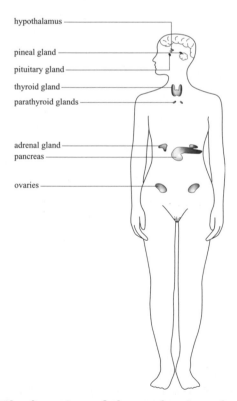

hypothalamus

pineal gland

pituitary gland

thyroid gland

parathyroid glands

adrenal gland

pancreas

ovaries

Figure 1.2 The location of the endocrine glands

How are the sex hormones produced?

There are three groups of sex hormones: the two female ones—oestrogen and progesterone—and a group of male hormones known as *androgens*. Having said that, women cannot produce any oestrogen without first making a male hormone. And men and women make both male and female hormones in order for their bodies to work correctly. It is the amounts of the particular male or female hormones within the body that differ between the genders. These three groups make up the family of sex hormones. A good analogy is musical instruments. The bassoon, oboe and clarinet are in the woodwind section of the orchestra and make a similar—but different—sound. Sex hormones are the same.

Androgen
The main male hormone or androgen is *testosterone*. The ovary produces much more testosterone than oestrogen, but then it converts some of this testosterone into oestrogen. If for some reason a woman was unable to make testosterone, then she could not produce any oestrogen. If a girl at puberty cannot produce any testosterone, then she cannot produce any oestradiol (a type of oestrogen—see below) and will remain sexually underdeveloped. Obviously men make a lot more testosterone than women, but men also make oestrogen. Interestingly, the average male produces more oestrogen than the average menopausal woman.

Myth: Women do not have any male hormones.
Fact: Women must be able to make testosterone, a male hormone, as without it they could not produce any oestrogen.

Usually the first hormonal event of puberty for a girl is the surge in a male hormone called *hormone dehydroepiandrosterone* (DHEA), made by the adrenal glands. The adrenals sit on top of the kidneys, one on each side. The inner part of the adrenals produces and releases adrenaline and noradrenaline, which prepare our bodies for 'flight or fight'. The outer part of the adrenals makes cortisone and DHEA, which is found in the bloodstream as DHEA sulphate (DHEAS). DHEA is itself inactive but is converted into other active hormones, such as testosterone. Rising levels of DHEA in a young girl stimulate the formation of armpit and pubic hair (called adrenarche).

In the bloodstream, a special liver-derived protein, called *sex hormone binding globulin* (SHBG), carries both testosterone and oestradiol. SHBG binds testosterone more strongly than oestradiol, so SHBG is normally saturated with testosterone rather than oestrogen. The hormone that is bound to SHBG is thought to be inactive and only the free hormone is biologically active. Many things can elevate or suppress SHBG, and this will affect free, biologically active testosterone levels (see Table 1.1). As we will discuss later, those with polycystic ovaries tend to have higher blood levels of free testosterone than those with normal ovaries, and this will make them prone to skin problems such as excess body hair and acne.

Oestrogen
As we saw earlier, oestrogen is responsible for breast development at puberty and the onset of menstruation. Oestrogen also thickens and

Table 1.1 Factors influencing levels of SHBG and free testosterone

	Effect on SHBG level	Effect on free testosterone
Oral oestrogen	Strongly increases	Lowers
Patch oestrogen	Minimal effect	No effect
Androgens	Suppresses	Increases
Insulin	Suppresses	Increases
Weight gain	Suppresses	Increases

stimulates the endometrium (the lining of the uterus). The ovaries produce most of the body's oestrogen, but many other tissues can also make this hormone, including fat, the breasts and the brain.

While most people have heard of oestrogen, the main female hormone, few realise there are three main types of oestrogen: *oestradiol, oestriol* and *oestrone*. Oestradiol is the most important oestrogen during a woman's reproductive years, and it is the most potent one. Oestriol is the main pregnancy oestrogen, and is produced by the placenta—which not only nourishes the baby, but is a major source of the female hormones that help maintain the pregnancy. After the menopause (the last period), when the ovaries stop working, the main oestrogen is oestrone and the main source of it is fat tissue. This is why overweight women tend to have an easier time at menopause and have stronger bones than those who are thin. The downside of this extra oestrogen from fat is that it seems to increase the risk of oestrogen-sensitive cancers such as breast and uterine cancer.

Myth: There is only one type of oestrogen.
Fact: Oestradiol is the main oestrogen of the reproductive years. During pregnancy, the most abundant oestrogen is oestriol, while after menopause oestrone is most prevalent.

Progesterone

Progesterone is mostly made after ovulation by the remains of the collapsed ovulatory follicle (the *corpus luteum*). It stops the oestrogen-induced growth of the uterus and tends to thin its lining if a woman does not conceive. (If a woman does conceive, progesterone helps maintain the pregnancy until the placenta starts producing the hormones necessary to do this job.) Progesterone also has effects on the breasts and uterus—broadly antagonising the effects of oestrogen.

Table 1.2 shows the main functions of the sex hormones.

Table 1.2 The main functions of the sex hormones

Oestrogen	Progesterone	Testosterone
Stimulates the breasts and the uterine lining	Tends to stimulate the breasts and thin the uterine lining, lightening periods	Converts into oestrogen
Maintains bone strength	May thin the vaginal skin	Stimulates hair growth in armpits and pubic area
Keeps the vaginal skin thick and moist	May have a positive effect on bone	Stimulates libido
Has an anti-depressant effect on the brain	Sedative, calming brain effect	Has a positive effect on the brain and bone

How are sex hormones regulated?

There are three main players that regulate sex hormones in both men and women: the pituitary, the hypothalamus and the testes or ovaries. In women, these three communicate with each other to fine-tune the hormones so that the body can be prepared for and carry a pregnancy.

The pituitary gland

The pituitary gland (see Figure 1.3) is situated behind the nose, at the bottom of the brain, suspended from the hypothalamus. It is very small, about the size of a thumbnail. It is the master gland that controls the development and functioning of important organs and systems throughout the body. It has two lobes, and it is the front part or 'anterior pituitary' that releases the hormones that regulate other glands in the body, including the thyroid, the adrenals and the ovaries in women, and the testes in men.

The hypothalamus

On top of the pituitary is a small area of the brain called the hypo-thalamus, which regulates many of the automatic functions of the

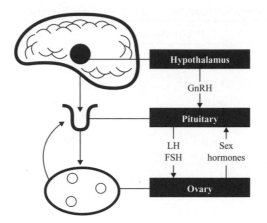

Figure 1.3 The hypothalamic–pituitary–ovarian axis

body such as temperature control. Within the hypothalamus is the *cyclic centre*, or *arcuate nucleus*, which regulates the pituitary's control of the ovaries. During the reproductive years, the cyclic centre fires a pulse of a hormone called *gonadotropin releasing hormone* (GnRH) every 90 minutes or so to stimulate the pituitary to release the two hormones that regulate the ovaries: *luteinising hormone* (LH) and *follicle stimulating hormone* (FSH). These two then act on the ovary to produce androgens and oestrogens and to stimulate ovulation. Other hormones such as activin can alter the action of FSH on the ovary. Activin stimulates pituitary FSH secretion, acts on the ovary to promote follicular growth and also affects insulin secretion.

The ovaries

Most of the fine-tuning of the menstrual cycle involves a dialogue between the ovaries and the pituitary. Using a 28-day cycle as an example (remember, a menstrual cycle ranges from 21 to 35 days), this is what usually happens:

Day 1   This is the first day of menstrual bleeding. The pituitary gland starts to release LH and FSH into the bloodstream to stimulate the ovaries. LH will act on the ovary to produce androgens, which will then convert into oestrogens under the influence of FSH. FSH will also cause the ovarian follicles to grow.

Day 7 A cluster of follicles on an ovary (usually only on one of the ovaries) can be seen using ultrasound scanning. A dominant follicle produces increasing amounts of oestrogen and another hormone called inhibin. The rising blood levels of these two hormones suppress FSH levels. LH levels are not affected as much as FSH.

Day 10 Blood FSH levels have dropped and, while these falling levels don't seem to affect the dominant follicle, the smaller follicles start to disappear.

Day 13 The dominant follicle has grown to about 20 millimetres (0.79 inches) in diameter (see Figure 1.4) and it signals the pituitary that it is ready to ovulate. This signal involves two hormones—very rapidly rising levels of oestradiol and progesterone. Either alone won't do it: both are needed. The pituitary then releases all its stored LH and FSH. Because FSH has been selectively suppressed for the days leading up

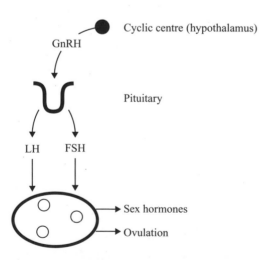

Figure 1.4 Control of follicular growth in the ovary

to this time, much more LH is released compared with FSH. This spike in blood levels of LH is called the *LH surge*. The LH surge does two things to the dominant follicle: it induces ovulation; and it switches on the egg to make it receptive to sperm.

Day 14 Ovulation takes place. A red bubble called a *stigma* forms on the surface of the follicle, which breaks down, allowing the egg to escape. It is then drawn into the nearby fallopian tube. The activated egg usually survives only a day or so and if it is not fertilised it will die. The remains of the follicle are converted into the corpus luteum, or 'yellow body'. The corpus luteum starts to produce large amounts of oestrogen and progesterone. As oestrogen and progesterone are essential for the maintenance of a pregnancy, the corpus luteum will continue to produce these essential hormones until the placenta takes over that job from about the eighth week of the pregnancy.

Day 21 If pregnancy does not occur, then the corpus luteum will start to die, and blood levels of oestrogen and progesterone will begin to fall.

Day 28 The top layer of the uterine lining needs oestrogen and progesterone to function. If these two fall to very low levels, then the endometrium dies and starts to slough off.

Day 1 Menstruation occurs. Most of the menstrual loss during the first two menstrual days is tissue from the endometrium; after that, most of the loss is bleeding from damaged uterine blood vessels.

Summary

Hormones play an important role in body function. Going back to the orchestra metaphor, think of hormones as the notes of the music. They need to be released by finely tuned glands (the instruments) so your body (the orchestra) can perform harmoniously. There are many types of hormones, including 'male' and 'female' ones. But note that both men and women must make both male and female hormones. Women need male hormones such as testosterone for their menstrual cycle to function normally. In fact, the ovaries produce more testosterone than oestrogen, although they convert some of this into oestrogen.

Problems occur when too much of a particular hormone is produced. For example, when testosterone is in the bloodstream, it is mostly attached to a carrier protein called SHBG. A small percentage of testosterone, however, is free. This is dissolved in blood, and is biologically active.

Excess free testosterone is like too many wrong notes being played. It can cause someone who is prone to develop skin problems such as excess body hair and acne to do so. As we will discuss later, those with PCOS tend to have higher blood levels of free testosterone than those with normal ovaries.

It is very important to distinguish between polycystic ovaries (PCO) and polycystic ovary syndrome (PCOS). It is thought that about one in four women, or 25 per cent, will be found to have PCO if they are screened on an ultrasound. If you are scanned and found to have PCO but have no symptoms, then you should consider yourself normal. As I will discuss in later chapters, problems such as irregular periods, acne and excess body hair that generally start around puberty are usually managed quite easily.

Around 5–7 per cent of all women will have PCOS, meaning they have two out of three of the following problems: polycystic ovaries; fewer than six periods per year; and/or blood or cosmetic evidence of excess male hormone production. As we will see later, long-term issues such as diabetes are more common for those with PCOS than for those who simply have polycystic ovaries and no symptoms. It is therefore vital that a correct diagnosis of PCOS is made, as this will determine how much—if any—treatment is required to manage symptoms.

Frequently asked questions

What's the difference between having PCO and PCOS?

It is quite likely that one in four women will be found to have PCO (polycystic ovaries) if their ovaries are scanned on an ultrasound. Most of these women, however, will have menstrual cycles every three to eight weeks. Women with PCOS (polycystic ovary syndrome) have polycystic ovaries and symptoms such as irregular periods and excess body hair. Those with PCOS are more likely to be at greater risk of more serious medical conditions, such as diabetes. All of these symptoms will be discussed in greater detail in Chapters 4 and 5.

Are women with PCO infertile?

No. Women with PCO whose menstrual cycles occur every three to eight weeks usually have little trouble conceiving. If they are having problems conceiving then they should have other fertility factors checked, such as the health of their fallopian tubes and their partner's sperm count.

What is a hormone?

Hormones are simply chemical messengers that coordinate bodily functions. They are produced in the glands of the body and are sent to other parts of the body to stimulate or inhibit a reaction. For example, the pituitary gland sends FSH to the ovaries to stimulate follicles to grow larger.

Do women make male hormones too?

Yes, it is essential for women to make male hormones. The ovaries produce testosterone, which is then converted into oestrogen. Thus a woman who can't make testosterone cannot make any oestrogen at all. Men produce both testosterone and oestrogen too, but men make a lot more testosterone than women do.

2
Looking for signs:
Polycystic ovaries and polycystic ovary syndrome diagnosed

As discussed in the previous chapter, polycystic ovaries (PCO) are common, affecting about 25 per cent of women during their reproductive years. Not all women who have PCO are aware of it, as it causes few problems. Some women, however, see a doctor because they have skin conditions such as acne, unwanted hair growth or menstrual problems. These could indicate PCO, or even PCOS, but they might also be due to some other factor, such as genetic inheritance or an unrelated hormonal imbalance.

Most medical authorities agree that PCO is present if there are more than twelve 2–9 millimetre (0.08–0.35 inch) follicles arranged around the periphery of the ovary in a 'pearl-necklace' pattern. Diagnosis of this can be difficult, however, because the difference between a 'normal' and a polycystic ovary is actually very subtle. An ovary is usually only about 3 centimetres (1.18 inches) long and a follicle (the fluid-filled structure on the ovary that contains an egg) may be only 2–6 millimetres (0.08–0.24 inches) in size. It is hard enough to see an ovary, let alone differentiate between a 'normal' and a polycystic one by looking at the pattern of the follicles. And then there's the added problem than an ovary is neatly tucked away deep inside the pelvic cavity.

How can doctors see an ovary?

When investigating for PCO, a doctor must be able to see the ovaries. They can do this by using abdominal ultrasound, vaginal ultrasound and/or laparoscopy.

Abdominal ultrasound

Ultrasound is a bit like a radar. Using soundwaves, a map is made of the area being scanned. The abdominal technique involves placing the ultrasound probe on the skin of the lower abdomen (over a full bladder). The sound beam must past through the skin, fat, muscle, bowel and bladder to find the ovary. This method is quick and pain-less (if a little uncomfortable), but because of all the layers the sound has to travel through, it can be difficult to see the ovary clearly. It is very easy to misdiagnose PCO using an abdominal ultrasound.

Vaginal ultrasound

The best ultrasonic way to pick up PCO, and by far the most common method, is to use a vaginal probe. A narrow ultrasound probe (about an inch wide) is covered with a protective sheath (to prevent patient-to-patient infections) and that sheath is then coated with a lubricating gel to aid insertion. The probe is gently passed into the vagina. As the ovaries and uterus are located at the top of the vagina, the vaginal probe can be placed virtually right onto the wall next to the ovary, producing high-quality pictures.

Because the probe is inserted into the vagina, this procedure may make some women anxious. I don't recommend the vaginal probe for women who have never been sexually active. In this instance, the probe may tear the hymen, causing pain and bleeding. For all other women, the procedure is perfectly safe. Indeed it should be pain-less—certainly no worse than having a pap smear.

Laparoscopy

Another common way for PCO to be discovered is during a laparoscopy. This surgical procedure involves the patient under-going a general anaesthetic (that is, being put to sleep) and then a small cut is made in the navel. An extremely small telescope is passed through this cut to allow the surgeon to easily view all the pelvic contents—the uterus, fallopian tubes, ovaries and so on.

Laparoscopy is usually performed when a doctor is investigating abnormalities of the abdominal or pelvic organs, such as investi-gating the fallopian tubes, ovaries or uterus for causes of infertility. It runs the same risks as all surgical procedures—damage to organs, infection and anaesthetic reactions—but the risk is minimal. It is not usually the first technique advised when diagnosing PCO because of the risks, but it provides an extremely good photographic-quality picture of the ovaries.

Do I have polycystic ovaries?

Once a doctor has a 'picture' of the ovaries, they need to make an assessment of what they see in order to diagnose PCO. When doing a laparoscopy, I like to use the top of the uterus as my ruler—the longest diameter of the ovary should be shorter than the top of the uterus. Polycystic ovaries are nearly always enlarged, often longer than the top of the uterus (see Figure 1.1). Also, polycystic ovaries have a smooth, thick outer lining and a pearly-white appear-ance. Often, but not always, the stroma—the middle part of the ovary that produces androgen—is also enlarged.

It is possible to have one polycystic ovary while the other is normal, but this is rare. When it does occur, a women's body seems to behave as though both ovaries are polycystic.

It's not PCO but it could be . . .

Sometimes an ovary may look almost like it might be polycystic, but it's not. An ovarian appearance that can be confused with PCO is that of *multifollicular ovaries*. These are a normal finding in girls going through puberty. The ovary is often enlarged and has numerous, different sized follicles (2–12 millimetres/0.08–0.47 inches) scattered throughout the ovary in no particular pattern.

Sometimes a patient can be convinced they have PCO, despite the image of the ovary indicating otherwise, because they feel pain in the pelvic area. PCO does not cause pain. It is more than likely that the patient has a cyst, and PCO has nothing to do with a cyst on the ovary. Normal follicles can normally grow up to 30 millimetres (1.18 inches), and the medical term 'cyst' is usually reserved for fluid-filled structures more than 30 millimetres (1.18 inches) in diameter. Most simple ovarian cysts disappear without any treatment. If a repeat scan shows that the cyst has persisted eight weeks later, then surgery is usually indicated.

> **Myth:** PCO are painful.
> **Fact:** PCO do not cause pain. Pain in the ovary could be from ovulation or from a cyst, which should usually clear up in time.

Do I have polycystic ovary syndrome?

Once a woman is diagnosed with PCO through ovarian scanning, she often automatically assumes that she has polycystic ovary syndrome.

PCOS is a complicated condition, which is usually only diagnosed when a patient presents with PCO and symptoms such as having fewer than six periods per year and/or excess body hair. We can also add to this diagnostic list one further tool: a blood test to measure hormone levels. So when a woman discovers that she has PCO, her doctor will need to examine her menstrual pattern, skin and hormone levels to confirm PCOS.

> When a woman discovers that she has PCO, her doctor will need to examine her menstrual pattern, skin and hormone levels to confirm PCOS.

Menstrual irregularities

The most common menstrual problem associated with PCOS is infrequent ovulations (fewer than six periods per year). However, it must be kept in mind that many other hormonal problems can cause irregular periods. Thus, if PCO is found during the investigation of irregular periods, this may or may not be the cause of the menstrual problem. It is not unusual for a woman who has PCO revealed through scanning to have another disorder, such as a thyroid problem, which may be the cause of the menstrual irregularity. All other possible causes of menstrual irregularity need to be excluded to confirm PCOS. There are a small number with PCOS who bleed fairly continually, which can be very distressing. Some swing between bouts of not menstruating, followed by continual bleeding for weeks on end. Causes of menstrual irregularities are discussed in more detail in Chapter 5.

Blood tests

In my experience, it is a common mistake to diagnose PCOS on the basis of a scan alone. It is imperative that the diagnosis always be confirmed by blood testing. The main reasons for performing blood tests is to exclude other causes of menstrual irregularity (see Chapter 5) in order to confirm that PCOS is the cause, and to check blood fat, glucose and insulin levels, which can be part of the syndrome. I have seen hundreds of women who in fact had premature menopause, not PCOS, and most of them suffered further because the correct diagnosis was delayed as it was thought that they were too young to be menopausal or they had a confusing and unclear ultrasound scan.

Every woman with menstrual irregularity should have some blood tests done. Ideally, bloods tests should be performed between days 1 and 7 of the cycle, before 10.00 a.m. and after an overnight fast (with water only permitted). This is because many hormones go up and down throughout the day and during the menstrual month. Eating affects blood fat, glucose and insulin levels.

The minimal tests I believe should be carried out are listed in Table 2.1.

Table 2.1 Basic blood tests for menstrual irregularities

Test	Reasoning
Pregnancy test	To exclude pregnancy
LH	Levels of 10–30 u/L (units per litre) suggest PCOS
FSH	Levels greater than 20 u/L (20 mu/mL) suggest menopause
TSH	To test for thyroid disease
Prolactin	To look for prolactin/pituitary problems

After eliminating all other causes of menstrual irregularity, a woman suspected of having PCOS will generally be given a further blood test to measure her hormone levels of testosterone, SHBG and the pituitary-released luteinising hormone (LH). The most common findings amongst women with PCOS are a slightly elevated level of testosterone, lowered levels of SHBG and elevated levels of LH. However, there is considerable overlap with these blood measurments between those with PCOS and those without. So it is advisable that other hormone levels be checked as well, including:

- FSH (to exclude early menopause);
- prolactin (for pituitary problems);
- TSH (for thyroid function);
- DHEAS;
- 17-hydroxyprogesterone (to check the adrenal glands).

I also always check the blood lipids (fats) and perform some measure of insulin function. Having said all this, no single blood test will be positive in every case of PCOS, but at least one of the following is nearly always the case:

- high LH;
- high total or free testosterone;
- low SHBG.

Table 2.2 Quick guide to what blood tests for PCOS might reveal

Blood test	What I expect in PCOS
LH	About half have an LH level greater than 10 u/L
FSH	Normal
TSH	Normal thyroid function
Prolactin	Normal
Testosterone	Upper limit of normal or raised
SHBG	Low half of normal or low
DHEAS	Normal or slightly raised
17-hydroxyprogesterone	Normal or slightly raised
Cholesterol	Might be raised
Triglycerides	Might be raised, indicating insulin resistance
Glucose	Normal usually; raised indicates diabetes
Insulin	Might be raised, indicating insulin resistance

My reasoning behind using blood tests to confirm a diagnosis of PCOS is best illustrated by the following patient stories.

Patient story: Suzie, 28 years old

Suzie came to see me as she was concerned about scalp hair loss. Her menstrual periods were regular but heavy, and an ultrasound scan had shown PCO. Her GP had ordered a hormone profile, which was normal, and in particular her thyroid function and male hormone levels were well within the normal range. As scalp hair loss is commonly caused by iron or zinc deficiency, I ordered a full blood count to check for anaemia, and for iron and zinc levels. I found that she was iron deficient and slightly anaemic. I treated her with iron tablets and the drug transexamic acid (trade name—Cyclokapron) to lighten her periods (see Chapter 5). Within six weeks, her scalp hair loss had returned to normal. In Suzie's case, the finding of PCO was a red herring: she did not have PCOS.

Myth: Scalp hair loss is usually due to PCOS.
Fact: Scalp hair loss may be due to an iron or zinc deficiency, and this possibility needs to be eliminated before PCOS is treated.

Patient story: Beth, 23 years old

When I first met Beth, she was concerned about significant excess body hair and the fact that she had only two periods a year. Her first period had been later than average, at age 16. Her local doctor had ordered an ultrasound scan which showed PCO. I asked Beth to fast overnight (no food after 10.00 p.m., although water is allowed) before her blood tests the following morning. The tests I ordered and Beth's results are given in Table 2.3, with the 'normal' range results for comparison.

Table 2.3 Beth's blood test results

Blood test	Beth's results	Normal range
LH, u/L	18	2–12
FSH, u/L (mu/mL)	4 (4)	2–12 (2–12)
Prolactin, ng/mL	8	<20
TSH, mu/L	1.7	0.4–5.0
Testosterone, nmol/L (ng/dL)	4 (115.3)	1.5–2.6 (43.2–74.9)
SHBG, nmol/L (ng/dL)	20 (0.58)	20–120 (0.58–3.46)
DHEAS, umol/L (ng/mL)	9 (3316.1)	<11 (4053.1)
17-hydroxyprogesterone, nmol/L (g/L)	2 (0.7)	<6 (2)
Glucose, mmol/L (mg/dL)	4.3 (77.5)	3.4–5.4 (61.3–97.3)
Fasting insulin, mu/L	35	<12
Cholesterol, mmol/L (mg/dL)	4.5 (173.7)	<5.5 (212.4)
Triglycerides, mmol/L (mg/dL)	2.8 (247.8)	<2.0 (177)

Not all pathologists use the same units and so it is always advisable to discuss your test results with your own doctor.

About 50 per cent of women with PCOS have a raised LH level when compared with the FSH level. Normally these two are found in similar amounts in blood (e.g. both would be around 4 to 6 units per litre). In some old textbooks, the diagnosis of PCOS required an LH to FSH ratio of at least three to one. Beth's LH/FSH ratio (calculated as 18 divided by 4) was 4.5 to 1. However, modern studies have found that no one hormone level will always locate the cases with PCOS. The best indicators are LH, testosterone and SHBG. Raised blood levels of LH and testosterone and low levels of SHBG are typical for PCOS. Each one will be positive for about half the PCOS cases. In Beth's case, all three fit the profile.

Some practitioners have found that a free androgen index (FAI) is a better indicator than testosterone levels alone. FAI is a measure of the biologically active free testosterone levels and is calculated by using the formula: testosterone × 100 divided by SHBG level. In Beth's case, this would be: 4 × 100 / 20 = 20. The normal range for FAI is usually less than 4.5. In my experience, the FAI will be positive in over 90 per cent of PCOS cases.

A raised fasting insulin level and/or raised triglyceride levels probably indicate insulin resistance, which will be discussed in detail in Chapter 6. Beth's fasting blood glucose level was normal, indicating that she was not diabetic, but she had raised fasting insulin and triglycerides, which is strongly suggestive of insulin resistance.

Beth had typical results for PCOS:

- Her LH level was much higher than her FSH—more than three times higher.
- Her LH level was high, her serum testosterone level was mildly elevated at 4 nmol/L (115.3 ng/dL) and her SHBG level was low at 20 nmol/L (0.58 ng/dL).
- Her FAI level was 20, much higher than the 4.5 normal range.
- The normal results for TSH, DHEAS and 17-hydroxyprogesterone exclude thyroid and adrenal problems.

FAI is a measure of the biologically active free testosterone levels and is calculated by using the formula: testosterone x 100 divided by SHBG level.

Patient story: Julie, 18 years old

Julie came to see me because she was having only two periods a year. Her first period occurred when she was twelve years old and they had been regular until about eighteen months before her visit to me. She also told me she had lost 10 kilograms (22 pounds) in weight for no apparent reason. Her ultrasound scan showed PCO. In my physical examination I found she had a very rapid, irregular pulse, but normal blood pressure. Her thyroid gland was smooth, but about twice the normal size. I ordered blood tests and they confirmed that she had an over-active thyroid. After treatment for her over-active thyroid, she regained 5 kilograms (11 pounds) and her menstrual cycle returned to normal. Once again, the scan finding of PCO was incidental; Julie did not have PCOS and therefore did not need any treatment for her PCO.

Summary

There are three ways a doctor can 'see' an ovary in order to diagnose PCO: through abdominal ultrasound, vaginal ultrasound or laparoscopy. Abdominal ultrasound does not provide as good a picture as vaginal ultrasound, and laparoscopy is a surgical procedure which is more invasive. I would firstly recommend a vaginal ultrasound to diagnose PCO.

It should be noted that a scan of the ovaries may not show PCO, but could show cysts on the ovaries or multifollicular ovaries. Both of these conditions should require no treatment. In fact, if a woman has PCO and her periods are regular, PCO should require no treatment.

However, between 5 to 7 per cent of the female population have PCOS—that is, PCO and symptoms such as irregular periods or excess body hair. However, amongst women having irregular periods, finding PCO on an ultrasound does not necessarily mean that this is the cause of the menstrual problem. In my opinion, all women having irregular periods should be carefully investigated to exclude other possible causes of the irregularity. To do this, I recommend full hormonal blood tests as these can exclude other causes such as thyroid imbalance.

Frequently asked questions

I have painful ovaries; does this mean I have PCO?

No. PCO does not normally cause pain. In fact, the PCO is not full of cysts. It is unfortunate that this condition is called polycystic ovaries, as it sounds like the ovaries are severely diseased, full of real cysts and painful. This name creates unnecessary fear for many women. The PCO has a ring of small, 2–9 millimetre (0.08–0.35 inch) follicles (not cysts) arranged in a 'pearl-necklace' pattern around the outer part of the ovary. Follicles are a normal part of the ovary and are not painful.

My doctor has asked me to have my ovaries scanned in case I have PCO. Will this hurt?

There are two main ways to scan the ovary: abdominal ultrasound and vaginal ultrasound. Abdominal ultrasound does not hurt at all, but doesn't necessarily provide a clear picture of the ovaries. Vaginal ultrasound does provide a clear picture of the ovaries, but it may cause a little discomfort—though no more than a pap smear.

I have irregular periods and excess hair and my vaginal scan showed PCO. Do I have PCOS or not?

You probably do have PCOS. The vaginal scan would provide a clear look at the ovaries, but you should have some blood tests performed to confirm a diagnosis of PCOS and to exclude other causes of menstrual irregularity. In my opinion, the minimum blood workup should measure LH, FSH, TSH, prolactin, testosterone (and SHBG), DHEAS, 17-hydroxyprogesterone, glucose (and insulin) and lipids. The blood should be collected before 10.00 a.m. in the morning after an overnight fast.

I have regular, heavy periods and have noticed a lot of scalp hair loss. Is PCOS the cause?

Probably not. You probably are iron deficient and I would recommend that you have a blood test to measure your blood count and iron level, and probably also your TSH level to rule out an under-active thyroid.

My periods have stopped and a scan shows PCO. Do I have PCOS?

You probably do have PCOS but it is essential that some blood tests be performed to confirm the diagnosis and exclude other causes of irregular periods.

3
Searching for answers:
Causes of polycystic ovary syndrome

Most women with either polycystic ovaries or PCOS are keen to know what caused it. The frustrating reality is that we don't know the cause for sure. There is probably more than one cause of PCOS, which has made finding the culprits very difficult, and in turn makes finding a single cure for all women unlikely. Broadly speaking, there are two possibilities: a genetic problem or an environmental cause (such as a dietary factor).

Are my genes to blame?

I have discussed the possible causes of PCOS with many experts, both in Australia and overseas. Most researchers believe that PCOS is probably caused by genetic factors because it tends to run in families. However, I will shortly outline the results of a twin study of PCOS which my research group performed. This study's outcomes dispute the hypothesis that PCOS is *usually* caused by genetic problems.

A number of studies have been undertaken that suggest genetics may play a part in developing the syndrome. In 1968, Dr Cooper and colleagues studied eighteen families in which the syndrome appeared to be inherited. He found that if a woman had PCOS, then around half of her sisters were also affected. Dr Cooper felt that these results suggested that PCOS may be inherited via a dominant genetic pattern. Normally we have two genes for different body functions—one from mum and one from dad. If a genetic condition is dominant, then just having one affected gene will cause the disease. When breast cancer runs in families, it is dominant—half the women get breast cancer and half don't. With a recessive genetic disorder, both genes need to be affected for the individual to have the problem. Cystic fibrosis is a common recessive disorder in most countries. An affected child has a double dose of the abnormal gene. Mum and dad are carriers of the disease—they have one affected gene and one normal gene. This means that they do not have the disease. Dr Cooper suggested that PCOS might be linked to the X chromosome in these families.

Dr Givens (1988) studied a group of women where PCOS seemed to run in the family. Again it was suggested that perhaps the problem lay on the female (X) chromosome. Dr Ferriman (Ferriman and Purdie, 1979), working in the United Kingdom, studied 381 women diagnosed with PCOS and found that just under 50 per cent of their female relatives had the syndrome as well—again suggesting a genetic inheritance.

In summary, most family studies have found that if a woman has PCOS, then her immediate female relatives have around a 50:50 chance of also having the syndrome. I must point out, though, that because a problem appears to 'run in the family', it does not necessarily mean the disorder is genetic. Families share common diet, exercise patterns, environmental factors and so on—tuberculosis used to run in families simply because family members coughed on each other.

Now that the human genome (our genetic code) has been identified, researchers are using gene technology to try to discover whether any genes might be linked to PCO and PCOS. To do this type of study properly, they need several hundred affected families.

To date, genetic studies have only focused on genes controlling oestrogen-androgen production, as well as insulin regulation, and no clear genetic link has yet been shown. The most promising link in this area relates to a protein called follistatin, an activin-binding protein. Activin is a hormone that stimulates pituitary FSH secretion, acts on the ovary to promote follicular growth and also affects insulin secretion.

A lot of family studies have shown that if a woman has PCOS, then her sisters and mother have a 50–80 per cent chance of having it too. This observation has convinced most researchers that PCOS is caused by genetic factors. This led my research team to perform a study of PCOS in twins, both identical and non-identical. The results were surprising.

A twin study of PCOS

This study was undertaken in the early 1990s as part of the PhD thesis of one of my students, Shayesteh Jahanfar. Most of this work was published in the journal *Fertility and Sterility* in 1995 (see Jahanfar et al., 1995). Australia has a register of twins that is kept in Melbourne. Using this wonderful research tool, Shayesteh wrote to 500 pairs of female-only twins living in Sydney. Thirty-four sets of twins took part in the study—nineteen pairs of identical twins and fifteen pairs of non-identical twins. A thorough medical history was taken, their height and weight were measured and they were examined for the presence of excess hair and acne. They also underwent ultrasound scanning to detect whether PCO was present, and a blood sample was collected.

If PCO is the result of a single gene problem, then it stands to reason that, amongst the identical twins, both should have the same type of ovaries—either both would be normal or both would have polycystic ovaries. Table 3.1 shows the preliminary results of the scanning. Using these results, we calculated a measure of inheritance called the Heritability Index (HI), and came up with a result of 0.28. As the HI approaches 1, genetic factors are more likely; if the HI is closer to 0, then environmental factors are more likely. In our study, the result of 0.28 made it unlikely that genetic factors had caused PCOS.

Table 3.1 Results of ultrasound scanning for PCO

	Identical twins	Non-identical twins
Both have normal ovaries	7 pairs	5 pairs
Both have polycystic ovaries	7 pairs	4 pairs
One twin has normal, the other has polycystic ovaries	5 pairs	6 pairs
Totals	19 pairs	15 pairs

Dr Nguyen, the statistician on the team, analysed the rest of the data and showed that most of the hormone measurements, such as testosterone, LH and FSH, were not under significant genetic control, but that BMI (body mass index, a measure of fatness or thinness—see Chapter 6), fasting insulin (see Chapter 6) and a hormone called androstanediol glucuronide (AG) were, at least in part, controlled by genetics. AG is produced by a skin enzyme called 5α-reductase. It correlates with the activity of this enzyme, which converts testosterone into the very potent male hormone, dihydrotestosterone (DHT). Raised blood levels of AG suggest that 5α-reductase activity is high, resulting in high skin levels of DHT, which can in turn cause acne or excess hair.

These results of the study would suggest it is very unlikely that PCOS is due to a single genetic problem. Our results are consistent with PCOS being the result of combined genetic and environmental problems, or possibly a genetic problem on the X chromosome (this is called 'a sex-linked' or an 'X-linked' disorder). The twin research model assumes that identical twins have identical genetics, but this may not always be the case.

> The twin study suggests that PCOS is likely to be the result of combined genetic and environmental factors. It is possible that, in some cases, the genetic problem lies on the X chromosome or could be the result of some intrauterine factor.

Women have two X sex chromosomes (males have a Y and an X), but they only use one at a time—usually about 50 per cent of the time for each, at which time the other one is resting. There have been case reports of twins where one has an X-linked genetic problem, but the identical co-twin doesn't. Genetic studies have shown that the affected twin has permanently switched on the 'bad' gene and the unaffected twin has the 'good' gene permanently switched on. Thus it is possible, in some PCOS cases, for there to be a genetic problem on the X chromosome of one twin, but not the other. Also, differences between identical and non-identical twins may not necessarily be the result of genetic mechanisms. In the womb, identical twins share their blood supply, as they are connected to one placenta. This may result in one twin being undernourished compared with the other. In other words, some intrauterine factors (see below) could cause some cases of PCOS.

The main implication of the genetic theories is that most researchers believe PCOS is permanent (because it is genetic), which means there are few long-term follow-up studies of the syndrome. My research team therefore also performed a study on patients of mine who had been diagnosed with PCOS at least five years previously. Most of these patients were treated with the contraceptive Pill. When we retested them, one-quarter no longer had PCOS. In other words, it seems that the syndrome can come and go.

When we retested those who were diagnosed as having PCOS more than five years ago, one-quarter no longer had PCOS. In other words, it seems that the syndrome can come and go.

Patient story: Ruth, 29 years old
Ruth has been a long-standing patient of mine with known PCOS. Her first period was late, at the age of sixteen years, and they were always irregular, coming once or twice a year. She starting taking the contraceptive Pill at age nineteen but had stopped (ten years later) as she was planning a pregnancy. When she stopped taking the Pill, her periods had become regular, on a monthly cycle. Ruth's ultrasound scan showed her ovaries were normal. It seemed that her PCOS had gone away.

Do I have too many male hormones?

Several researchers have suggested that excess androgens can convert a normal ovary into a polycystic ovary. Some years ago, Dr Amirika (Amirika et al., 1986) found that female-to-male transsexuals given testosterone developed PCOS. Thus it would seem that, at least in some cases, there might have been an initial androgenic 'insult' that changed normal ovaries into polycystic ones. In turn, these altered ovaries exacerbate the problem if they continue to produce excess male hormones. It is even possible that the androgenic insult might occur while the foetus is developing inside the uterus (see below) or at puberty, or it might be the result of excessive testosterone exposure, or an adrenal condition such as 21-hydroxylase deficiency or Cushing's syndrome.

Professor Yen (1980), an American PCOS expert, suggested over twenty years ago that the polycystic ovary was the result of an exaggerated surge of adrenal hormones. Certainly, most of my patients date their problems from puberty, which is when the first hormone event is a surge of male hormones (see Chapter 1). It is usually a surge of the adrenal androgen DHEA which is responsible for the production of pubic and armpit hair (adrenarche).

It is also well described that most women with an inherited adrenal androgen problem (e.g. 21-hydroxylase deficiency, which I will describe in detail in Chapter 5) have PCO. Most women with cortisol over-production, the so-called 'Cushing's syndrome', have PCO as well. In my opinion, Professor Yen's suggestion that an exaggerated surge of adrenal androgens may trigger PCOS is an attractive theory and is probably one of the many ways in which a young woman might develop this common problem.

Is it my brain hormones?

A high blood level of the pituitary hormone LH is found very commonly amongst women with PCOS. In part this may be due to a lack of ovulations, since both oestrogen and progesterone inhibit LH (and FSH) in the luteal phase of the cycle. However, some with regular ovulations have high LH levels, suggesting that in some cases of PCOS there may be either a pituitary problem or a very subtle problem with the control loop between the ovary and the pituitary. Some animal studies have suggested that a female pituitary can be 'masculinised' if exposed to high male hormone levels in the intrauterine or perinatal period. This results in an increased release of LH, which in turn would stimulate the ovary to over-produce androgens—creating a vicious circle. How relevant this may be in humans is hard to say. I tend to place this sort of information in the 'just interesting' category.

Did it happen before I was born?

Pregnancy is associated with a modest rise in testosterone levels, especially in the first twelve weeks when the foetus's ovaries are developing. The placenta has a large amount of the enzyme aromatase, which should convert the androgen into oestrogen, but interestingly there have been case reports of female foetuses being masculinised by androgen-secreting ovarian tumours. This at least raises the possibility that a female foetus's ovaries could be altered inside the uterus by excessive male hormones.

It has also been suggested by a number of researchers that an insulin resistance (IR) problem may start in the uterus. The hypothesis here is that, if the mother is malnourished, then perhaps she 'signals' to her foetus that times are tough. The foetus becomes IR because IR confers survival advantages in a famine (for a fuller discussion on IR, see Chapter 6). If this were true, then small, growth-retarded babies should have the highest rates of diabetes and PCOS. Dr Laitinen (2003) studied 2007 women and found that, rather than skinny, growth-retarded babies having the highest risk of PCOS, the converse was the case. Fat, overdue babies seem to have the highest risk of PCOS (Laitinen, 2003). For me, it makes a lot of sense that mum might 'communicate' with her foetus in utero. However, at the moment it is not clear how this might happen.

Was it something I ate?

In the twin study discussed above, we found that some identical twins had different ovary types. This made us rethink the causes of PCOS. As some family studies have shown that PCOS runs strongly in families, we wondered whether perhaps it wasn't genetic; rather, other factors common in families might cause PCOS. The research group came up with at least two strong possibilities: eating disorders or something in the food itself.

Eating disorders

Shayesteh Jahanfar, the student who conducted the twin study for her PhD in the early 1990s, reviewed medical literature for evidence relating eating disorders to PCO. The literature suggested that around 20 per cent of young women suffer from an eating disorder. Dr McClusky and colleagues (1992) used a questionnaire called BITE (Bulimia Investigation Test Edinburgh) to investigate cases of PCOS. When they asked women to complete this, they found that over a third of women with PCOS showed evidence of an eating disorder. Shayesteh performed her own study to see whether she could verify the Scottish study (see Jahanfar and Eden, 1996). She sent the BITE questionnaire to 94 female-only twin pairs. She found that women diagnosed with PCO were six times more likely to have a mild eating disorder than those with normal ovaries. She also found that eating disorders were under strong genetic control but that the severity of the disorder was determined by environmental factors. Thus it is possible that an eating disorder such as anorexia or bulimia may in some way change normal ovaries into the polycystic type. Or perhaps certain diets may affect the function of the ovaries.

Hidden in the food

At around the same time as Shayesteh was conducting her questionnaire study, I started reading in the veterinary literature about a condition in sheep called 'clover disease'. This is a common problem in Australia because of our soils. Farmers plant clover to help enrich the soil. Legumes, such as clover and beans, take nitrogen out of the atmosphere and fix it in the soil, which is a great benefit for the animals and the farmer. However, clovers also make a plant chemical called phytoestrogens, or 'plant oestrogens'. These chemicals are properly called isoflavones.

If the sheep are fed exclusively on the clover, they consume too much isoflavone and develop clover disease, which renders the sheep infertile. This disease closely resembles human PCOS. I have had several long discussions with veterinary experts about clover disease and the similarities with PCOS are striking. They are summarised in Table 3.2.

Table 3.2 Sheep clover disease and human PCOS

	Sheep clover disease	Human PCOS
Ovaries	Polycystic	Polycystic
LH levels	High	High
Androgen levels	Not measured yet	High
Effect on ovulation	Suppression	Suppression
Skin effects	Virilised	Excess hair and acne
Uterine lining	Thick	Thick

I noted that several papers on clover disease commented on the fact that the sheep were virilised, or masculinised. (In humans, this means growing hair in excess in places that men do, such as on the face as a beard.) But how do you tell whether a sheep is virilised? After all, a sheep is already hairy. I rang an Australian expert on clover disease, Dr Norm Adams, who told me that the entrance of a sheep's vagina closes over when there is a high male hormone level. Clover disease doesn't affect all sheep in the same way, though. There seems to be a genetic vulnerability. We also know that it isn't the plant isoflavone that is the problem, but rather a phyto-estrogen called 'equol', which is produced by the friendly germs in the sheep's gut.

Applying this story to the human situation, it is important to keep in mind that these sheep eat only clover, and they eat lots of it—we rarely eat only one type of food. My research group has already had a preliminary look at phytoestrogens and human PCOS, but there is a lot more work needed in this area. My working hy-pothesis is that perhaps some women produce 'bad' phytoestrogens, either because of a genetic vulnerability or because of their particular gut flora (which we get from our immediate environment, like our family, through the foods we eat). I have also seen cases where a healthy diet seemed to cause PCOS.

Patient story: Philippa, 25 years old
Philippa came to see me with a very interesting story. Her periods were regular when she ate her normal high-fat, high-carbohydrate, junk-food diet. However, whenever she ate healthy foods for a while (meaning lots of fruit and vegetables, whole grains, etc.), her periods stopped. I first met Philippa during one of her 'healthy eating' phases. She had not menstruated for four months. Her blood tests showed typical PCOS. Clearly something in her 'healthy diet' was suppressing her periods. We were not able to identify the problem food.

The more you weigh

We have already touched on the importance of weight maintenance for those with PCOS. Weight gain tends to aggravate the symptoms of PCOS, so weight control is clearly an important aspect of managing the problems. One convenient method for estimating fatness or thinness is body mass index (BMI). It is calculated using the formula BMI = weight in kilograms divided by height in metres, squared (i.e. BMI = kg/m^2). Normal BMI ranges from 20 to 25 kg/m^2. If your BMI is over 25 then you are overweight; a BMI of under 20 suggests you are a bit underweight.

BMI = weight/height squared (kg/m^2). Normal BMI ranges from 20–25 kg/m^2. If your BMI is over 25 then you are overweight; a BMI of under 20 suggests you are a bit underweight.

Does insulin resistance affect PCOS?

Over the past decade, research has suggested that a condition known as insulin resistance (IR) plays a central role in the cause of some women having PCOS. Most reviews on this subject (for example, Dr Tsilchorozidou and colleagues in 2004 and Professor Dunaif in 1997) suggest that between 30 and 60 per cent of women with PCOS have evidence of IR.

Women affected with IR have raised blood insulin levels and an exaggerated blood insulin response to a carbohydrate load. High insulin levels have been shown to stimulate the ovaries to produce more testosterone and lower blood levels of SHBG, resulting in high free, biologically active levels of testosterone. There is also some evidence that high insulin levels are also responsible for the high levels of LH found in around half the women with PCOS.

Increasing weight gain aggravates IR, so blood insulin levels rise further—which in turn leads to high levels of free testosterone, resulting in decreased ovulations and often a worsening in excess hair or acne. Chapter 6 discusses IR in more detail, examining what is it, how it can be diagnosed and how it can be prevented or cured.

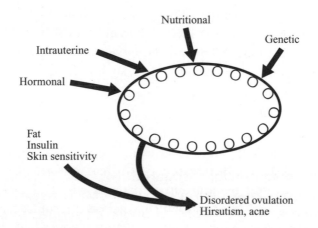

Figure 3.1 Causes of PCO

Summary

I have long suspected that there is no one cause of PCOS, but rather several. In some patients, there clearly seems to be a genetic factor operating, but our twin study indicates that it is unlikely that most cases of PCOS are due to a single genetic problem. Some women may have their ovaries affected by an androgenic insult inside the uterus, at puberty or even in adult life. There is a strong link between PCOS and eating disorders, and this observation, combined with the extraordinary story of the 'sheep clover' disease, strongly suggest that diet plays a key role in some cases—not just in terms of how often a woman with PCO menstruates, but also in developing the disorder in the first place. It is also clear that PCOS is not always permanent, but rather can come and go.

Frequently asked questions

Does PCO run in families?

Yes, studies have shown that 50–80 per cent of the direct relatives of women with PCOS have at least PCO when scanned. This doesn't necessarily mean that PCO is caused by genetics, however, as many other factors can be similar in families, such as diet.

Is PCOS permanent?

There are remarkably few long-term studies that examine this important question. My research group has performed one small study: we reinvestigated a group of patients who had PCOS more than five years ago. Most of them had taken the contraceptive Pill for at least two years. One in four of them no longer had clinical or ultrasound evidence of PCOS.

Does diet have a role in PCOS?

There is no doubt in my mind that diet plays an important role in PCOS. Our research, together with other findings, has shown a strong link between PCOS and eating disorders such as anorexia and bulimia. In sheep, a diet high in phytoestrogens causes a disease called 'clover disease'. This seems to be the sheep equivalent of PCOS. The sheep become virilised and stop ovulating. As I will discuss in later chapters, a diet high in fat and carbohydrate and weight gain seem to aggravate the symptoms of PCOS.

4
Scratching below the surface:
Skin and hair symptoms

Around half the women with PCO have a skin problem, usually in the form of excess hair or acne, although a minority will suffer scalp hair thinning or loss. Two studies discussed below, 'A thousand cases of PCOS' (Eden and Warren, 1999) and 'The resistant acne study' (Eden, 1991), illustrate several important points. First, PCO is commonly found amongst women with acne, especially severe acne. Second, there seems to be a relationship between excess body hair and blood androgen levels, but little or no relationship between the severity of the acne and blood androgen levels. Third, hormonal therapies are effective in the treatment of these conditions, irrespective of whether or not there is an identifiable hormonal problem.

Why does hair grow or not grow?

Hair is made of keratin, a protein. Every strand of hair will grow longer and longer over several months as keratin is released into the root of the hair. Hair grows from the sebaceous follicle, or the root, and each follicle has a cycle of growth (see Figure 4.1). Scalp hair follicles may have a growth phase of two to five years, whereas the short hairs on the back of the hands may only have a growth phase of two months. Eventually the growth phase stops then, after a period of time, the hair falls out. The follicle then rests for a short period before growing another hair. Hair follicles contain androgen and oestrogen receptors as well as enzymes to produce male and female hormones.

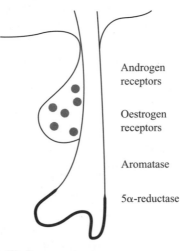

Androgen
receptors

Oestrogen
receptors

Aromatase

5α-reductase

Figure 4.1 Hair follicle

There are two main types of hairs—vellus and terminal. Vellus hairs are fine and lightly pigmented, and usually not noticed. Vellus hairs resemble 'peach-fuzz' and are produced by small hair follicles. On the other hand, terminal hairs are dark and thick and are produced by large follicles. The larger the follicle, the thicker or coarser the hair. Terminal hairs are normally found in the armpits and pubic area and, in men, on the face, shoulders, chest and back. Some areas of the body, such as the scalp, eyebrows and eyelashes, do not need androgens to grow. However, androgen excess can contribute to a type of 'male-pattern' baldness (receding frontal hair line and thinning on the top of the scalp rather than on the sides) in some women.

Too much hair

Most women absolutely hate excess body hair. Hirsutism refers to the presence of terminal hair in women (and children). Depending on how one defines the severity of the problem, and of course the racial group studied, between 12 and 50 per cent of women suffer from hirsutism. And virtually all of them want to do something about it. For some women, it is the facial hair that is most disturbing. Apart from the cosmetic viewpoint, some women think they are turning into a man and they often believe there is nothing they can do to reverse the hair problem. As you will read below, there are a number of treatments that will help to control this symptom.

Myth: Some women with hirsutism think that they are turning into a man.
Fact: You can't be female without making male hormones.

Hirsutism in women may be defined as the presence of terminal hair in areas where it is more usual for men to grow hair—the face, shoulders, chest and back. Each hair follicle has receptors to both oestrogen and androgen, but the main culprit in this story is not the androgen testosterone, but rather a more potent male hormone called dihydrotestosterone (DHT). The skin takes up testosterone from the bloodstream and converts it in the hair follicle into DHT, under the influence of an enzyme called 5α-reductase. As I discussed in the previous chapter, our twin study of PCOS showed that the activity of this enzyme is virtually entirely genetically controlled. This explains why some races are not hairy (e.g. the Chinese) but others are very hairy (e.g. the Greeks).

5α-reductase is also found in the prostate gland. With the current research interest in prostate cancer, it is likely that there will be some spin-off treatments for androgen-excess disorders. For example, the drug cyproterone acetate (CPA), sold under the brand name Androcur, inhibits 5α-reductase and suppresses ovarian (or testicular) testosterone production. CPA also blocks the androgen receptor and so this 'three-way action' makes it a very successful therapy for prostate cancer in men and androgen excess hair disorders in women.

It is not known why this male hormone stimulates terminal hair on the face, but causes loss of hair on the scalp. It is clear from the many research studies undertaken, however, that hair follicles are not all the same in terms of their responsiveness to hormones. Therefore, any treatment needs to be carefully thought through so the correct hormone is treated and the right dosage is given.

> Hair follicles are not all the same in terms of their responsiveness to hormones.

A thousand cases of PCOS

In 1999, Dr Peter Warren (the Director of Ultrasound at the Royal Hospital for Women in Sydney) and I published a review of 1019 consecutive cases (seen between July 1989 and December 1994) of PCOS, all diagnosed by ultrasound. We assessed all the women for hirsutism and sorted them into three groups: mild or no excess hair; moderate excess hair; and severe excess hair. A total of 347 of the women (35 per cent) had significant excess body hair. For all the women, we checked their body mass index (or BMI— see Chapter 6) and their levels of testosterone, SHBG and DHEAS. Then we averaged the results and summarised them as shown in Table 4.1.

As you read Table 4.1 from left to right, it can be seen that the women with the worst excess hair problem had a higher BMI—that is, they were heavier—and had higher testosterone levels than the

Table 4.1 Average results for women with excess body hair

	Mild or no excess hair	Moderate excess hair	Severe excess hair
BMI	23	27	27
Testosterone, nmol/L (ng/dL)	1.6 (46.1)	2.2 (63.4)	2.4 (69.2)
SHBG, nmol/L (ng/dL)	47 (1.36)	39 (1.12)	32 (0.92)
DHEAS, umol/L (ng/mL)	6.9 (2542.4)	7.6 (2800.3)	8.2 (3021.4)

women with less or no hair problem. The higher testosterone and lower SHBG levels resulted in even higher free testosterone levels. Interestingly, bloods levels of the adrenal androgen, DHEAS, were also higher in those with the worst excess hair problem.

Why is my face breaking out all the time?

Many factors contribute to the development of acne. These include the amount of oil (sebum) in the skin, a blockage of pores, abnormal skin germs or inflammation. Severe cases of acne often run in families. Oestrogen seems to reduce oil production in skin, whereas androgen enlarges the oil-producing glands, which produce more sebum. A germ called *Priopionibacterium acnes* (or *P. acnes* for short) digests the sebum, making it thicker and blocking oil glands, as well as producing chemicals that cause inflammation.

In the 'A thousand cases of PCOS' study discussed above, we checked the patients for acne and found that the presence and/or severity of acne did not correlate with any blood hormone level. Most researchers have found the same thing—the severity of excess body hair correlates well with blood androgen levels (the higher the testosterone, the worse the excess hair), but this does not seem to be the case for acne. The reasons for this are not clear, but may in part be explained by the observation that acne is affected by many non-hormonal factors, as already discussed.

The resistant acne study

In 1991, I published the results of a study in the *Medical Journal of Australia* that I called 'the resistant acne study' (see Eden, 1991). This study involved 30 women with very severe acne whose response to known treatment was unusual. All 30 women failed to respond to two courses of isotretinoin, an oral medication that causes the skin to peel. It is normally a very effective treatment for acne—one six-month course cures over 80 per cent of cases of severe acne. The fact that these women had failed to respond to two courses of the drug meant that they had really nasty, unresponsive acne.

For this study, I used an acne scoring system devised by Dr Marynick (Marynick et al., 1983) for measuring severe acne. This system counts spots greater than 5 millimetres (0.20 inches) in size, usually on the face, chest and back, which are rated as shown in Table 4.2. A score of 4 means there are more than twenty 5 millimetre (0.20 inch) acne spots in that area.

Table 4.2 The Marynick acne scoring system

Grade of acne	Lesions more than 5 mm (0.20 inches)
0	0
1	1–5
2	6–10
3	11–20
4	more than 20

The ultrasound scans of the 30 women in the study showed that nineteen had PCO and eleven did not. Blood tests were undertaken and the results were averaged for each of the two groups. These are summarised in Table 4.3.

Table 4.3 Average blood results

	Normal ovaries	Polycystic ovaries
Testosterone, nmol/L (ng/dL)	1.0 (28.8)	1.4 (40.3)
SHBG, nmol/L (ng/dL)	57 (1.64)	35 (1.01)
FAI	1.4	5
DHEAS, umol/L (ng/mL)	5 (1842.3)	8 (2947.7)

Those with PCO on the scan had higher testosterone and DHEAS levels, lower SHBG results and so higher FAIs than those with scan-normal ovaries. But once again, the severity of the acne did not correlate with the blood levels of any of the hormones.

All the women in this study were then treated with Cyproterone acetate (trade name—Androcur), taking 100 milligrams per day for ten days with 21 days of oestrogen (ethinyl oestradiol, or EE, 50 mcg). The regimen involved taking both Androcur and EE for the first ten days, followed by eleven days of EE alone, then a seven-day break. Androcur can also be taken with the contraceptive Pill (such as Diane-35). Typically, two 50 milligram tablets of Androcur are taken with the first ten active contraceptive Pills. Androcur is a type of progestin and an androgen-blocker. This dual action makes Androcur very, very useful. As a progestin, it thins the lining of the uterus (making the periods light) and protects the uterus from cancerous change. As an androgen-blocker, it is a very effective treatment for acne and hirsutism.

Using the Marynick acne scoring system Table 4.4 shows the average results (i.e. each woman on average rated 4 on the Marynick scoring system at the beginning, and 0 at the end of six months). The range of the results is shown in brackets.

All the women improved dramatically with the treatment, irrespective of whether they had PCO. As the table shows, most of them were much better within six weeks. I have found Androcur to be a very effective treatment for acne; however, it can cause some weight gain, fluid retention and breast soreness.

Table 4.4 The effect of Androcur treatment on average (range) acne scores

Acne score	Normal ovaries	Polycystic ovaries
Initial	4 (1–7)	4 (1–7)
6 weeks	1 (0–4)	1 (0–3)
12 weeks	0 (0–0)	0 (1–0)
6 months	0 (0–0)	0 (0–0)

Myth: There are no really effective treatments for severe acne.
Fact: Hormonal therapies, such as Cyproterone acetate, are effective irrespective of whether or not there is an identifiable hormonal problem such as PCO. Isotretinoin is also useful.

Do hormones affect the skin and hair?

Sex hormones can profoundly affect the look, texture and health of your skin. In general, skin loves oestrogen. It promotes fluid retention, filling out wrinkles. Oestrogen also stimulates the skin to produce more collagen and elastin, which helps the skin maintain its thickness—collagen and elastin bind skin cells together to maintain the thickness. Normal ageing, sun exposure, cigarette smoking and lack of oestrogen all contribute to the thinning of skin over the years.

All sex hormones tend to promote fluid retention, which is part of the reason so many women suffer from premenstrual fluid retention. You may have noticed that at different times of your cycle your skin condition changes. This is because oestradiol and testosterone surge on the day of ovulation, then seven days later both oestradiol and progesterone levels peak, falling again just before your period. Testosterone and oestrogen also have marked effects on your hair follicles and sweat glands. Table 4.5 shows the effects of these hormones on your skin.

Men produce at least ten times more testosterone than women, which is why they have more facial and body hair. Men also have a higher risk of acne and scalp hair thinning than women because of these high testosterone levels. With age, all men lose hair, usually beginning on both sides of the frontal hairline and on the top of the scalp, with less loss on the sides of the head. Some women with high androgen levels also develop 'male-pattern' baldness.

How skin reacts to male hormones is under strong genetic control. Baldness tends to run in families—the men in an affected family may be bald by their thirties, whereas the women in the same family usually notice significant hair loss around ten to twenty years later, and it is usually not as severe as for the men. It is quite rare for a woman to go completely bald. There is at least one study (Ferriman and Purdie, 1979) showing a link between baldness in the men and PCOS in the women of the same family. Scalp hair loss may also be a sign of an under-active thyroid, or of an iron or zinc deficiency, malnutrition, sickness or stress.

Table 4.5 The effects of oestrogen and testosterone on skin

Oestrogen	Testosterone
Promotes water retention	Promotes water retention
Stimulates collagen and elastin	
Reduces oil production	Increases oil production
Improves acne	Aggravates acne
Blocks the effects of testosterone on skin and hair	Causes the hair follicles to produce thick, dark hair
Promotes normal scalp hair growth	Scalp hair thinning, receding frontal hairline

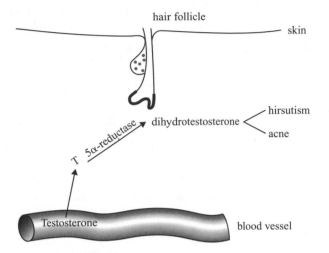

Figure 4.2 The effect of testosterone on skin

Myth: All hair loss is due to PCOS.
Fact: Scalp hair loss may also be a sign of an underactive thyroid, or of an iron or zinc deficiency, malnutrition, sickness or stress.

Which hormonal tests should I have?

If you suspect you have a high level of androgen causing an excess hair problem, then it is worthwhile getting your doctor to check:

- blood levels for male hormones—usually testosterone and SHBG (and also calculate an FAI) for ovarian androgens;
- DHEAS and 17-hydroxyprogesterone to check the adrenal gland functions;
- blood test to check thyroid function (TSH).

About a third to half of those with PCOS have a mildly raised level of DHEAS, the adrenal androgen. If blood levels of DHEAS are very high, this may be due to a hormone-secreting lump in the adrenal, called an adenoma. These can be seen using a CT scan or MRI scan. A raised level of 17-hydroxyprogesterone suggests a genetic adrenal hormone problem called 'congenital adrenal hyperplasia', although this can also be due to an adrenal adenoma. Both of these will be discussed in more detail in the next chapter.

If your menstrual cycle is irregular, then you should also have the levels of these hormones checked:

- LH;
- FSH;
- prolactin.

If scalp hair loss is a problem, then your blood tests should also include:

- full blood count (looking for anaemia);
- iron studies;
- serum zinc level.

The blood test for iron is very accurate and one component of this test, a serum ferritin, reflects the body's iron stores. If the serum ferritin level is low, then the body has exhausted its iron stores and anaemia is sure to follow. I see many women who have scalp hair loss that is due to iron deficiency, even though they have a normal blood count. If the iron deficiency is not treated, these women will eventually become anaemic. In my experience, scalp hair loss often occurs before anaemia and the iron deficiency is usually due to heavy periods. The blood test for zinc is not as accurate as the iron test.

How do you treat hair and skin problems?

There are a number of ways to treat hair and skin problems successfully. Depending on the severity of your conditions, you might want to discuss the following options with your doctor.

Physical methods of hair removal

Removing the unwanted hair is the main method women use to control hirsutism. Among the many physical methods for removing hair, there are simpler methods and more complicated ones. These include:

- *Shaving.* Simply shaving the hair with a razor or an electric shaver is quick, simple and cheap. However, it needs to be done often (usually daily) and the hair tends to grow back as stubble (and can look like a 'five-o'clock shadow').
- *Plucking.* Tweezers are used to grasp the hair and pull it out root and all (ouch!). It is cheap and simple, and the effect lasts longer than shaving. However, it is painful and can cause redness, and sometimes even a mild infection (folliculitis). It can also stimulate the hair follicle so it's probably best to avoid it.
- *Waxing.* This is usually done using hot wax. After application to the area, it cools and hardens. The set wax is then removed (ouch again!) with the hair and its root. Many of my patients use a mixture of beeswax, sugar and honey that seems to work really well, without too much pain. The effect lasts several weeks. On the negative side, waxes can irritate the skin, causing redness and inflammation.
- *Bleaching.* The hair is not removed, but rather is bleached using hydrogen peroxide. This method is quite useful for mild facial and arm hair. However, it can really only be used for fine hairs. Like waxing, bleaches can irritate the skin.
- *Depilatory creams.* These chemically dissolve the hair. Depilatory creams are often used on the legs and bikini line, but skin

irritation is common, especially when used on the face. The effect seems to last longer than shaving, but not as long as waxes.
* *Laser hair removal.* In the past ten years there has been an increasing vogue for using laser for hair removal. This is much more expensive than electrolysis—often ten times more—and the results are not always permanent. The procedure should be painless, and the effects are long-lasting and in some cases permanent. However, there are many women who have spent thousands of dollars on laser hair removal yet still have a substantial amount of excess body hair. The side-effects of laser removal include redness, blistering of the skin, excess pigmentation in the treated area or even white patches in dark-skinned women, indicating a loss of skin pigmentation.
* *Electrolysis.* Electrolysis is an established method of permanent hair removal, but its effectiveness is dependent upon the expertise of the operator. A tiny wire is passed down into the follicle to burn the base of the follicle, which destroys the hair-producing root. The side-effects of this method can include inflammation of the follicle, pigmentation of the treated area and even scarring. I usually recommend that a test area be done before performing electrolysis on the face to avoid further problems.

Physical methods for dealing with acne scarring

Unfortunately, some with severe acne develop deep scars and pits, which are especially noticeable on their face. Dermabrasion, dermaplaning and chemical peels can really improve this situation. Plastic surgeons or some dermatologists usually perform the first two procedures. Doctors or beauty therapists can perform chemical peels.

Plastic surgery for scarring
Dermabrasion and dermaplaning can really help improve the look of acne-scarred skin. These are performed under a general anaes-

thetic. Dermabrasion involves scraping away the top layers of skin, usually with a small wire brush or sometimes a diamond-tipped burr. Dermaplaning removes some of the top layers of skin. The idea is to 'smooth out' the skin. The website of the American Society of Plastic Surgeons (www.plasticsurgery.org) has some excellent information about these two techniques. Side-effects are uncommon, but include pigmentation, whiteheads, scarring and infection. If you are considering this type of plastic surgery, have a good talk to your local doctor and be sure that you are referred to a qualified plastic surgeon or dermatologist.

Chemical peels

If you've ever been sunburnt, you'll have some idea how a chemical peel works. The skin is induced to peel using a variety of chemicals (fruit acids, glycolic acid, lactic acid, phenol). The old skin comes away and the new skin that emerges is smoother than the old. Many types of acne respond to peels. A lot of my patients have used hormonal therapies in combination with 'a peel' to dramatically improve their acne. After the peeling agent is applied, the skin tingles for around ten minutes and then stinging often follows. Depending on the type of chemical used, the skin peeling can go on for a couple of days, or even a couple of weeks. The skin is often red for some days. Long-term side-effects are uncommon, but include scarring and abnormal pigmentation. The American Academy of Dermatology's website (www.aad.org) is an excellent resource for this topic.

Dermatological approaches

Mild acne can be successfully treated with topical peeling agents (e.g. those containing retinoic acid) or facial peels using fruit acids or glycolic acid. Topical antibiotics are also useful. The two most popular types contain small amounts of either clindamycin (about 1 per cent) or erythromycin (about 2 per cent).

Moderately severe acne can be treated with oral antibiotics such as tetracyclines, erythromycin or trimethoprim. The most severe cases are usually offered oral isotretinoin, which can only be prescribed by dermatologists. It is given as a six-month course and during this time it often produces marked peeling and skin redness. A potentially serious side-effect is that it can cause foetal abnormalities if pregnancy occurs while taking the drug, but there are no lingering problems in this area once the course is completed. During the treatment it commonly causes marked drying of the eyes, mouth and nose, so moisturisers are required.

You may be wondering why anyone would take this drug, but a six-month course of isotretinoin cures around 80 per cent of cases of severe acne. For such affected people, it is often seen as a 'miracle drug'.

> A six-month course of isotretinoin cures around 80 per cent of cases of severe acne. For such affected people, it is often seen as a 'miracle drug'.

The oral contraceptive Pill

Those women who develop excess body hair usually start to notice it between fourteen and eighteen years of age, unless they are taking the contraceptive Pill. There are many brands of the Pill available, including:

- Diane-35;
- Marvelon;
- Femoden-ED;
- Minulet;
- Yasmin;
- Trioden-ED;

- Tri-Minulet;
- Microgynon 20; and
- Loette.

The Pill prevents the development of hirsutism and acne. Some contraceptive Pills offer particularly good treatments for excess hair and acne because they contain a small dose of a male-hormone blocker (see below). But most contraceptive Pills are useful therapies for both acne and excess hair as they suppress the ovarian-derived excess testosterone and stimulate SHBG levels, resulting in very low free testosterone levels in the body.

Myth: The contraceptive Pill causes excess body and facial hair.
Fact: The Pill is a good treatment for hirsutism as it suppresses the ovaries, lowering testosterone levels.

Clinical trials have shown that virtually all contraceptive Pills offer good treatments for acne, but some are better than others. Two of them, Diane-35 and Yasmin, both contain a small amount of a synthetic progestin, which is actually a male-hormone blocker. (Progestins are a synthetic form of progesterone, which is the female hormone that lightens the periods and protects the uterus against cancer.) But some women notice mood changes such as irritability and even depression on the Pill, and these usually relate to the progestins. For example, if a woman became depressed on Triphasil, then she should avoid all Pills containing the progestin levonorgestrel. This includes Microgynon 20, 30 and 50, Triquilar and Loette.

Some women notice mood changes such as irritability and even depression on the Pill, and these usually relate to the progestin component.

The most studied contraceptive Pill for androgen excess disorders is Diane-35. If 100 women with acne take Diane-35, then after twelve months of use, 90 will be much improved. By three months, only about 30 per cent will be better. Clinical trials have shown that Diane-35 is also useful for mild to moderate cases of excess body hair, but that it may take one to two years to see the full impact of this treatment. Yasmin is particularly useful for women who have suffered from progestin side-effects such as fluid retention, depression or weight gain after using other contraceptive Pills.

Patient story: Claire, 27 years old
Claire came to see me because she had severe persistent acne and scan evidence of PCO. However, her menstrual cycle was regular and she did not have any evidence of excess body hair or scalp hair loss. Her hormone profile was normal. She had seen a dermatologist, who had offered her isotretinoin, but she was reticent to take it because of side-effects. She was taking Microgynon 20 for contraception and had noticed that her skin had improved by about 50 per cent since she had begun to use it. I suggested she swap from Microgynon 20 to Diane-35 and that she use topical clindamycin (a topical antibiotic) lotion for one to two months. I saw her again four months later and her acne had cleared considerably.

Problems with the contraceptive Pill
The contraceptive Pill seems to attract a lot of unfair press. There are side-effects, and these can relate to either the oestrogen or progestin component. It is usually a matter of finding the right balance between the two components. The oestrogen part can cause nausea and breast soreness, which usually disappear after one to three months. (Nausea was a much greater problem years ago when the original Pill had a very high-dose preparation, but it can still ocur with today's lower dose Pills.) Taking the tablet with food can

minimise this side-effect. Most of the Pill's side-effects relate to the progestin component, and these include fluid retention, mood swings and weight gain—but they are much less common with the newer Pills.

Around a quarter of women starting modern contraceptive Pills notice irregular menstrual bleeding in the first month or two—this is normal and usually settles by the third or fourth month of therapy. Stopping and starting different brands of the Pill when you are trialling them can induce irregular bleeding. It is prudent to try a particular Pill for at least three months before changing to another. Antibiotics, some vitamins and some drugs used to treat epilepsy and asthma may interfere with the absorption of the Pill, causing spotting or leading to its failure to work—in other words, you could become pregnant. If you miss a Pill, it should be taken when remembered and the next one taken on its correct day. In this case, you should use another method of contraception (e.g. condoms) until the next period occurs to avoid unwanted pregnancy.

> Stopping and starting different brands of the Pill when you are trialling them can induce irregular bleeding. It is prudent to try a particular Pill for at least three months before changing to another.

Patient story: Kerry, 32 years old
Kerry had been on the Triphasil contraceptive Pill for two years and felt very depressed while taking it. Microgynon 20 had produced a similar effect on her mood. When she stopped the Pill, her mood lifted within two weeks. I suggested that she try Yasmin and she has been fine ever since.

Cyproterone acetate

Cyproterone acetate (CPA), as mentioned above, is an extremely useful drug for the management of severe androgen-excess disorders. It is an androgen-blocker—which means it suppresses the ovarian production of testosterone—and it is a progestin, so it protects the uterus against cancer and lightens menstrual periods. Diane-35 contains 2 milligrams of CPA, but it is also available in the form of a drug known as Androcur. All levels of acne and excess body hair respond to this drug.

CPA is usually given with oestrogens, and it is my usual practice to combine it with Diane-35. The full dose is two 50 milligram tablets given with the first ten active Pills of Diane-35. Contraceptive Pills come in packets of 21 active tablets, and some then have seven days of inactive tablets as a reminder to have a seven-day break from the medication (see Figure 4.3). The CPA tablets are taken with the first ten active contraceptive Pills.

Even severe acne usually improves within three months of this therapy. Hirsutism takes longer to clear, but by the fourth month of treatment the hair is usually thinner, lighter and physically removed more easily. A severe case of hirsutism usually takes twelve to 24 months of treatment to see a marked improvement.

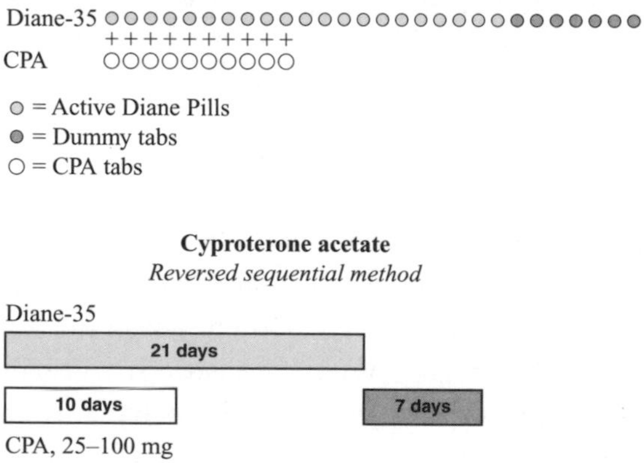

Diane-35 ○○○○○○○○○○○○○○○○○○○○○○○○○○●●●●●●●●
CPA   +++++++++
      ○○○○○○○○○○

○ = Active Diane Pills
● = Dummy tabs
○ = CPA tabs

Cyproterone acetate
Reversed sequential method

Diane-35

21 days

| 10 days | | 7 days |

CPA, 25–100 mg

Figure 4.3 The contraceptive Pill and CPA

This drug is usually very well tolerated by most patients, but side-effects may include weight gain, fatigue, breast tenderness, nausea, depression and headaches. The two cases that follow illustrate the usefulness of this drug.

Patient story: Margie, 32 years old

Margie came to see me because of severe persistent acne. She had already tried two courses of isotretinoin but the acne had returned. Her menstrual cycle was normal and monthly, and while she had evidence of PCO through ultrasound scanning, her hormone levels were normal. When I examined her, she had severe pustular acne virtually all over her face, back and chest. I prescribed Diane-35 and CPA and her periods lightened considerably to just one day of light-brown discharge, which is normal on this type of treatment.

I saw Margie again three months later and all her acne was gone. After six months of therapy I referred her to a plastic surgeon for dermabrasion to reduce the scarring caused by the acne. After twelve months of combined therapy, her skin looked normal so I asked her to reduce the amount of CPA she was taking but to continue with Diane-35. Three months later, I asked her to reduce the CPA again. Two years after our initial consultation, Margie had normal skin and was only taking Diane-35.

Patient story: Melinda, 18 years old

Melinda came to see me because of irregular periods and moderate excess body hair. Her scan and blood tests were consistent with her having PCOS. I put her on Diane-35 and six months later the excess hair was only slightly improved. I then asked her to take CPA as well. Nine months later, Melinda's excess hair problem had all but disappeared, so she stopped the CPA but remained on the Diane-35 to keep the problem under control.

Both of these cases illustrate an important point. The skin's sensitivity to androgens is under strong genetic control. Once a good result has been obtained with CPA, it is stopped but the contraceptive Pill is continued to keep the skin problem under control. If the Pill is stopped too, then the excess hair or acne usually comes back. Thus most women who have been successfully treated with CPA need to stay on a contraceptive Pill to control their skin problem, at least until they are ready to come off the Pill to have a baby.

Spironolactone

This is a diuretic, a tablet designed to get rid of excess fluid. It was discovered by accident to also be a male-hormone blocker. Many years ago, it was given to men with fluid problems and some of them started to lose their facial hair. Like CPA, spironolactone is a very useful medicine for treating androgen-excess disorders. It reduces testosterone production but also blocks 5α-reductase activity in skin. Most clinical studies have focused on using spironolactone to treat excess body hair. Male-pattern baldness in women may also respond to a contraceptive Pill with CPA or spironolactone. Clinical trials have suggested that about half of such cases respond to either of these drugs, although it may take a long time to see an effect.

The usual starting dose of spironolactone is 100 milligrams daily. It works best when used with a contraceptive Pill, but spironolactone can also be used on its own. It is very safe, but can cause breast soreness, nausea and dizziness (as it may lower blood pressure slightly). Most diuretics cause the body to lose some potassium, but not spironolactone. If there is a history of kidney problems or similar medical complications, then I usually recommend checking blood sodium and potassium levels every three to six months. For most healthy young women, this is not necessary. It is vital to remember that spironolactone is *not* a contraceptive. If a woman conceives whilst taking this drug, a male foetus may be exposed to a feminising drug. Theoretically, this might have an adverse effect on his sexual development.

Patient story: Trudy, 14 years old

Trudy had severe excess hair due to PCOS, but I was reticent to give her the contraceptive Pill because of her age. (There is an enormous amount of information about the Pill given to women between the ages of 16 and 50 years, but very little information concerning its use in girls under the age of 16.) I suggested she try spironolactone alone, without a contraceptive Pill, but I warned her that one in four women using spironolactone alone developed frequent periods (two to three a month). She tolerated the treatment very well, with no side-effects, and by the time she reached 16 her excess hair problem had disappeared. I then offered Trudy either a lower dose of spironolactone daily or a low-dose contraceptive Pill to keep the problem under control. She chose to take the lower dose of spironolactone.

Patient story: Sandra, 18 years old

Sandra came to me with severe excess hair. She had scan-PCO. Sandra responded well to CPA and Diane-35, but her weight had increased by 6 kilograms (13 pounds). I suggested she swap to Yasmin and spironolactone, which she tolerated without any problems. A year later, the excess hair problem was much improved, and she was back to her normal weight. I then asked her to stop the spironolactone and stay on the Yasmin.

Topical eflornithine

As is so often the case in medicine, a drug that is invented for one disease is often found to be useful for others. Eflornithine was synthesised as a potential cancer treatment and is used to treat African sleeping sickness! Eflornithine blocks an enzyme (ornithine decarboxylase) that is essential for the growth of hair. Topical eflonithine must be used twice daily and scientific studies have shown that less than 1 per cent of the drug is absorbed into the body. If the treatment is stopped, the hair regrows. Clinical trials (e.g. Barman Balfour and McClellan, 2001) have shown that, after 24 weeks of treatment, 58 per cent of those treated with topical eflornithine were judged to be 'clinical successes' or 'improved', compared with only 34 per cent in the placebo group. Side-effects include redness (1–2 per cent), acne (20 per cent, but the placebo group had the same rate of acne), and burning or tingling (15 per cent, compared with only 5 per cent in the placebo group).

Minoxidil

This active ingredient was invented to lower blood pressure and found to be useful for treating scalp hair loss. Dermatologists often prescribe Minoxidil lotion (2–5 per cent solution) for scalp hair thinning and loss. It is used topically on the scalp twice daily and appears to work by opening up scalp blood vessels and improving the function of the hair follicles. Once again, the treatment may have to be used for twelve months before any improvement is seen. It can sometimes cause scalp itch and dryness. In many countries it is sold over the counter.

Iron and zinc supplements

If iron deficiency is diagnosed, then your doctor will probably recommend that you take an iron supplement for at least three months before your blood is tested again for iron stores. If your periods are heavy, then your doctor should consider treatment for that too (see Chapter 5). In cases of scalp hair loss, it is a good idea to try a zinc supplement containing 20–50 milligrams of zinc, with one tablet taken daily for at least two months as a trial. If the scalp hair loss is due to either iron or zinc deficiency, the hair loss should slow within four to six weeks.

There are a couple of practical points that should be made about iron and zinc supplements. Iron is fairly poorly absorbed into the body. Acid and vitamin C help, so it is a good idea to take your iron supplement with some citrus juice. The body absorbs iron, zinc and copper through a similar gut mechanism. Thus, if a high dose of zinc—say, more than 50 milligrams daily—is taken for several months, then theoretically the body may become deficient in iron and/or copper. Also, iron and zinc supplements probably shouldn't be taken together, but rather separated by several hours. If both are needed, it is best to take one in the morning and the other in the evening.

Natural therapies for hirsutism or acne

Many of my patients who suffer from acne find that some natural products such as dilute tea-tree oil applied to the affected skin can be very helpful. There is no doubt that tea-tree oil is an excellent anti-septic. Oral herbals that are often tried for acne and hirsutism include saw palmetto, agnus castus and red clover. Unfortunately, there is little scientific evidence that these herbals help these skin conditions. Two of the best herbal textbooks around, *Principles and Practice of Phytotherapy* (Bone, 2000) and *Rational Phytotherapy* (Schulz et al., 2001), had only minimal sections on acne and excess hair.

Summary

Around 10 per cent of women of reproductive age will have signifi-cant excess body hair. Most just put up with it or simply remove it. Many are unaware that simple effective treatments are available. I offer the contraceptive Pill with CPA or spironolactone to most of my patients with excess body hair. After twelve months of therapy, more than 90 per cent have improved. Once the problem has significantly improved, most only need to stay on a low-dose contraceptive Pill to keep the problem under control, although some will choose to take a low dose of spironolactone instead. Acne also responds very well to these treatments.

Physical therapies such as chemical peels, dermabrasion and dermaplaning can really help reduce scarring caused by acne. Unwanted hair can be removed via a variety of methods ranging from waxing to laser therapy.

Those suffering from scalp hair loss need to be investigated for iron, zinc and thyroid hormone deficiency, and for androgen excess problems. Those who are iron or zinc deficient respond promptly to supplements: the hair dropping slows, usually within a month. Around half of those with scalp hair loss due to androgen excess will respond to anti-androgen therapy.

Frequently asked questions

Doesn't the contraceptive Pill cause excess body and facial hair?

This is a common urban myth. The Pill is a good treatment for hirsutism as it is designed to suppress the ovaries, so it lowers testosterone levels. The oestrogen component raises blood levels of SHBG and so bioactive free testosterone levels are substantially lowered by the Pill. Clinically, the Pill usually stops the hair getting worse, but to get rid of excess body hair an anti-androgen is needed. The two commonly used anti-androgens are spironolactone and Cyproterone acetate.

I have really bad acne. Can hormonal treatments help?

Yes. Hormonal treatments seem to work well for acne, whether or not an androgen-excess disorder is found. A good starting point is a contraceptive Pill. Mild cases often respond even to low-dose Pills, such as Loette or Microgynon 20. More severe cases are best treated with Diane-35 combined with CPA. Once the acne has cleared, then the dosage of CPA can be reduced or even stopped. Usually the Pill is continued to keep the problem under control. If the acne is angry looking and red, often topical or oral antibiotics can be really helpful too.

Which is the best contraceptive Pill for acne?

All contraceptive Pills are useful for acne. Diane-35, Marvelon or Yasmin are probably the best ones at the moment.

I've heard that removing facial hair makes the problem worse. Is that true?

No. Treatments such as waxing, creams, electrolysis and probably laser actually slow the hair growth. Plucking might stimulate the hair follicle and is probably best avoided.

5
Counting the days:
Menstrual irregularities

As discussed earlier, a woman's menstrual cycle is usually 28 days long, but it can be as short as 21 or as long as 45 days. The length of the cycle is important, as the egg in the follicle needs a certain amount of time to mature. At ovulation, the dominant follicle releases the egg and the remains of the ovulatory follicle become the corpus luteum ('yellow body'). The corpus luteum produces large amounts of oestrogen and progesterone and, if pregnancy does not occur, it dies after fourteen days.

From a medical point of view, doctors do not usually investigate infrequent periods unless they come less often than six times a year, or frequent periods unless they are coming less than every 21 days, or bleeding is longer than seven days. Finding out what is causing your menstrual irregularities is important so the correct treatment can be used. Some will have scan evidence of PCO and be aware that something else is going on. Thus all women who are experiencing irregular periods will require some tests. In my opinion, a minimum work-up would include a pregnancy test and blood levels of LH, FSH, prolactin and TSH. The blood sample is best taken before 10.00 a.m., as some hormones have a daily rhythm (e.g. prolactin is lowest in the morning and highest in the evening). Women with excess body hair, acne or scalp hair loss should also have their male hormone levels—testosterone, DHEAS, SHBG and 17-hydroxyprogesterone—checked as well. Any abnormal tests should be repeated to ensure they are accurate, and not caused by stress or some other single event.

Ultrasound scanning can also provide useful information. Women with pituitary problems or true early menopause will have small, inactive ovaries with few follicles visible. A small uterus with a thin lining suggests a low-oestrogen state. A thick uterine lining is often found in conjunction with the polycystic pattern. Finally, women with low-oestrogen state anovulation probably should have a bone density test performed to make sure that they are not developing osteoporosis.

There are a number of specific reasons why women with PCOS have menstrual problems, and a number of reasons that may have nothing to do with PCOS. At any one time, between 5 and 10 per cent of women are experiencing menstrual irregularity and about 1 per cent will have very infrequent periods (that is fewer than two periods a year). This section discusses how PCOS can affect your cycle, and looks at other causes of menstrual irregularity. It also takes a look at fertility issues, as this is a major concern for many women.

Why do many women with PCOS have a menstrual problem?

Menstrual problems are common for those with PCOS. But in order to be diagnosed with PCOS, other causes of menstrual irregularity must be excluded. If you suffer from PCOS, you may find your cycle is shorter or much longer than those of other women. You may also find your periods are heavier than what is considered normal. In my experience, more than 90 per cent of the women

I see with PCOS tell me that their periods become more irregular as they gain weight. This is not surprising, as SHBG levels fall with increasing weight—probably because of increasing blood levels of insulin, the sugar hormone. (Chapter 7 discusses insulin in more detail.) As SHBG levels fall, free testosterone levels will rise, acting as a brake on the menstrual cycle and aggravating any existing skin problem such as acne or excess body hair.

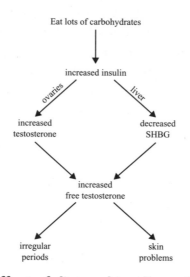

Figure 5.1 The effect of diet and insulin on free testosterone

Chapter 1 explained why testosterone is an essential hormone for a woman to be female: the ovaries convert some testosterone into oestradiol (the main type of oestrogen). Thus, if a young woman could not make any testosterone, she would not go through puberty. She could not make any oestrogen at all, which would mean that she could not develop breasts, have periods or conceive. That's why producing adequate amounts of testosterone is an essential part of being a woman.

However, like all our hormones, blood testosterone levels need to be maintained within a certain range for normal bodily function. Too

Myth: Women only make female hormones.
Fact: Producing adequate amounts of testosterone is an essential part of being female.

little testosterone—such as when a woman is anorexic or menopausal—and the periods stop. Too much testosterone and the periods can also cease, as happens in PCOS. Many with PCOS have insulin resistance (see Chapter 7). If these women have a high carbohydrate meal, they over-produce insulin, which in turn stimulates the ovaries to make testosterone, as well as suppressing liver production of SHBG. These effects will increase bio-active, free testosterone levels (see Figure 5.1). There are exceptions to this observation of increasing weight leading to fewer periods, however. A small number of women with PCOS are thin, even pathologically thin. Researchers and clinicians often refer to these women as 'thin PCOS'. Some of these women have an overt genetic factor operating; others do not.

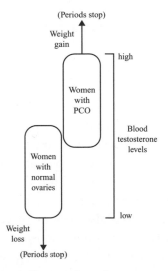

Figure 5.2 The effect of weight change on testosterone and menstruation

The 'thousand cases of PCOS' study revisited

This study was discussed in Chapter 4 in relation to skin problems. It also revealed much information about the menstrual disorders associated with PCOS. To recap, between July 1989 and December 1994, I saw 1019 women who had evidence of PCO on ultrasound scanning. Table 5.1 summarises the menstrual regularity of these women and Table 5.2 summarises the clinical and hormonal data for the group.

Table 5.1 Menstrual regularity of women in the 'thousand cases of PCOS' research

Period regularity	Number of women
Fewer than 3 periods a year	255 (25%)
3–10 periods a year	464 (45.5%)
11–15 periods a year	275 (27%)
More than 15 periods a year	25 (2.5%)

Table 5.2 shows that the women with very infrequent periods were more likely to have a late first period and be overweight than those experiencing regular periods. They also had higher androgen and LH levels than their normally cycling counterparts. This confirms the relationship between BMI and the hormonal problems in PCOS. Increasing BMI was associated with a worsening hormone profile and symptoms. This is also true in my clinical practice—most women with PCOS find that their menstrual (and skin) problems worsen as they gain weight. Conversely, weight loss tends to normalise SHBG and free testosterone levels, and restores the menstrual irregularity.

Table 5.2 Clinical and hormonal data (expressed as averages) from the 'thousand cases of PCOS' research

Periods per year	11–15	3–10	2 or less	*Significant difference?
Age at first period (years)	12.7	13.0	13.4	Yes
Weight (calculated as BMI, kg/m²)	23.7	24.8	24.8	No
LH, u/L	4.6	6.9	7.9	Yes
FSH, u/L (mu/mL)	5.1 (5.1)	5.8 (5.8)	5.7 (5.7)	No
Testosterone, nmol/L (ng/dL)	1.6 (46.1)	1.8 (51.9)	2.2 (63.4)	Yes
SHBG, nmol/L (ng/dL)	42.0 (1.21)	44.0 (1.27)	33.0 (0.95)	Yes
DHEAS, umol/L (ng/mL)	7.1 (2616.1)	7.4 (2726.6)	7.5 (2763.4)	No

* Statistical tests were applied to these results to determine whether these differences were real or likely to be by chance. In science, if the chance of a result occurring is calculated to be less than 1 in 20 (expressed in scientific papers as 'p<0.05'), then it is deemed likely that differences observed are real.

Most women with PCOS find that their menstrual (and skin) problems worsen as they gain weight. Conversely, weight loss tends to normalise SHBG and free testosterone levels and restores the menstrual irregularity.

On the other hand . . .

There are, however, exceptions to all rules. One of my patients, who weighed 140 kilograms (309 pounds), had severe excess body hair and markedly raised blood androgen levels, yet she had perfectly regular menstrual periods. I have also seen many women who are thin but have PCOS. These exceptions to the rule remind me that we do not know the whole story about PCOS.

Patient story: Karen, 14 years old

Karen came to see me with her mother and it was obvious she had PCOS. She had severe excess body hair and had not yet had her first period. However, she was thin—her BMI was 18 (normal is 20–25). Yet her blood profile confirmed PCOS. She also had five first-degree relatives with late-onset (Type 2) diabetes (indicative of insulin resistance). Karen's fasting insulin level was over 500 mu/L (normal is usually 12 mu/L) and her fasting blood glucose was just into the diabetic range at 6.5 mmol/L or 117.1 mg/dL (normal range 3.4–5.4 mmol/L or 61.3–97.3 mg/dL). Clearly, in Karen's case there was an insulin problem running strongly in her family. In her case, genetics was more important than her weight.

Myth: Amongst those with PCOS, only women with a higher than average weight will suffer from menstrual irregularities.
Fact: Thin women can also suffer PCOS-caused menstrual irregularities; however, the number of these women is much smaller—only 5–10 per cent.

There is another exception to consider as well. Around 1–2 per cent of women with PCOS seem to bleed continuously. Some may bleed for a month for so, have a week off, then bleed again. Others may go for six months without their periods and then they bleed continually for months on end. Ultrasound scanning usually shows that these women have a thick lining of the uterus (endometrium), which fails to shed completely. Because they have usually failed to ovulate, they have incurred a continual secretion of oestrogen without the protective effect of progesterone—no progesterone is made by the dying follicle and it is progesterone that thins the endometrium. When they do finally have a period, it can be very heavy and prolonged. Sometimes the period is so severe that the woman can end up in hospital. The hospital doctor may think that a miscarriage is occurring—after all, she is 'overdue' and is bleeding heavily. A sensitive blood pregnancy test is usually negative, and the heavy bleeding is simply due to a greatly thickened uterine lining. This very unpleasant scenario could have been prevented by using a course of progestin tablets (or even a contraceptive Pill) to thin the uterine lining.

Patient story: Barbara, 35 years old

Barbara was taken to casualty by a friend because she was bleeding very heavily, passing clots and feeling faint. Barbara was known to have PCOS and she had always had irregular periods, about two to three a year. At this time she had not menstruated for six months, but had been bleeding heavily for two weeks. A pregnancy test was negative. The doctor found she was anaemic and she was admitted to hospital for a blood transfusion and a dilation and curettage (D&C) to stop the bleeding. A D&C involves the neck of the uterus being stretched (or dilated) so the lining of the uterus can be scraped (or curetted) out under a light anaesthetic. Barbara was sent home after two days with a prescription for a contraceptive Pill to prevent further episodes of such heavy bleeding.

Most women with PCOS will find that weight gain worsens the frequency of their periods. Around 5–10 per cent of those diagnosed with PCOS will be thin. And around 1–2 per cent of women with PCOS will suffer from bouts of heavy continual bleeding. It is possible to have PCO confirmed by scanning, only to discover that another condition is causing the menstrual irregularity. An ultrasound finding of PCO does not necessarily mean that PCOS is the cause of the menstrual problem. Many conditions can mimic PCOS, so all women with menstrual irregularity should have some blood tests done to exclude these other problems.

It is possible to have PCO confirmed by scanning, only to discover that another condition is causing the menstrual irregularity.

What else causes menstrual irregularities?

Sometimes an underlying condition other than PCOS may cause menstrual problems. The main concern from a doctor's perspective will be that the affected woman will either be oestrogen-deficient, and therefore at risk of osteoporosis, or will be producing unopposed oestrogen that can stimulate the lining of the uterus to thicken, producing very heavy periods and increasing the risk of cancer of the uterus.

If a woman is lacking in oestrogen, then she may be at risk of osteoporosis. Most women with PCOS who are having infrequent periods are not at risk of developing osteoporosis, but may be at risk of premalignant uterine changes.

The usual hormonal causes of irregular periods are:

- stress;
- prolactin problems;
- anorexia nervosa;
- hypothalamic-pituitary disease;
- premature menopause;

Myth: All women with menstrual irregularities have PCOS.
Fact: Many conditions can cause menstrual irregularities, so women suffering from this condition should have blood tests to exclude other causes before treating PCOS.

- ovarian problems;
- thyroid disease;
- adrenal problems;
- uterine problems.

Stress

The cyclic centre within the hypothalamus is connected to many parts of the brain and receives information from many hormones. If the brain receives a signal that there is some significant stress on the body, it switches off the cyclic centre, causing ovulation to stop. This is a protective mechanism as it isn't a good time to fall pregnant—the major biological impetus of the reproductive cycle. It is common for young women sitting their final exams to stop menstruating during that stressful time. Blood testing at the time usually reveals low or low to normal levels of LH and FSH because the cyclic centre has been suppressed and pituitary drive has been reduced. Low levels of LH and FSH result in low blood levels of oestradiol. Such women inevitably find that their periods return after exam time.

Patient story: Jessie, 27 years old
Jessie's baby was stillborn. After this traumatic experience she lost 7 kilograms (15 pounds) of weight over six months. Twelve months after the baby was lost, her periods still had not returned. I tested her blood and her results are shown in Table 5.3.

Her LH and FSH levels were in the low to normal range and the other results were normal. This suggested her cyclic centre had switched down. After counselling, she gained some weight and her periods slowly returned.

Table 5.3 Jessie's blood test results

Hormone result	Jessie's results	Normal range
Pregnancy test	Negative	
LH, u/L	1	2–12
FSH, u/L (mu/mL)	2 (2)	2–12 (2–12)
Prolactin, ng/mL	5	< 20
TSH	2.5	0.4–5.0
Testosterone, nmol/L (ng/dL)	0.5 (14.4)	1.5–2.6 (43.2–74.9)

Prolactin problems

Prolactin is another hormone made by the anterior pituitary. Its main function is to stimulate the production of breast milk. A baby suckling on the breast releases more prolactin, which keeps the milk flowing. This excess prolactin turns off the hypothalamic cyclic centre so ovarian function is suppressed. This is why breastfeeding mothers usually do not have menstrual periods for four to six months or so after giving birth. This is perfectly normal. But there are certain situations where a non-lactating woman makes too much prolactin, causing her periods to stop and possibly causing a milky discharge from the breasts. The important factors that elevate prolactin are:

- stress;
- drugs—antidepressants, antinauseants, drugs for schizophrenia;
- an under-active thyroid;
- chest wall trauma or stimulation;
- pituitary adenoma;
- non-prolactin-secreting pituitary tumours, which are rare.

If a raised prolactin level is detected in a blood test, the test should always be repeated to confirm there is a problem because prolactin is a stress hormone and it undergoes a daily rhythm. It is lowest in the morning and so a blood sample for prolactin should always be collected before 10.00 a.m. A persistently raised prolactin could be associated with low or normal LH and FSH levels, since prolactin suppresses the cyclic centre and the pituitary release of these two hormones. Thyroid function should always be checked too, since an under-active thyroid can induce high prolactin levels. The pituitary can also be scanned using either a CT or MRI scanning. These scans sometimes show an adenoma of the pituitary. 'Adenoma' means simply lump. In most cases of raised prolactin levels, the pituitary adenoma is tiny—less than 10 millimetres (0.39 inches) (microadenoma)—and only rarely larger (macroadenoma). There are a number of treatments for prolactin problems, depending on the underlying cause. The most commonly used are one of two drugs— bromocriptine or cabergoline. They are highly effective, lowering blood prolactin levels, shrinking a pituitary adenoma (if present) and restoring the cycle.

Patient story: Melissa, 28 years old

Melissa had been suffering from a prolactin problem for years and did not menstruate unless she took prescribed drugs (cabergoline). Her untreated prolactin level was around 5000 mu/L (the normal range is less than 400 mu/L). An MRI scan showed a 3 millimetre (0.12 inch) microadenoma. She took two carbergoline tablets a week and her prolactin levels returned to normal. Melissa soon fell pregnant and then breastfed her baby for six months. Her periods returned while she was breastfeeding, and when she finished breastfeeding, her pro-lactin level and MRI scan were found to be completely normal. During her pregnancy, her high levels of oestrogen stimulated her prolactin cells, so they became 'hooked' on oestrogen. Following the birth of the baby, her oestrogen levels fell dramatically, but the tiny pituitary adenoma had 'died', which cured her problem.

Anorexia nervosa

Eating disorders are common in young women. These women can have a distorted body image, thinking they are overweight when any objective measure of their body composition indicates they are underweight. They often swing between starving themselves and bingeing, before inducing vomiting—a condition known as bulimia. Some become so ill they have to be admitted to hospital to be force-fed.

A BMI less than 19.1 (the normal range is 20–25) is associated with an increased risk of menstrual irregularity. From the reproductive point of view, these women nearly always stop menstruating because their cyclic centre slows and can even stop. They often 'go backwards through puberty'. First their periods stop, and if they continue to lose weight their breasts shrink and they can even lose pubic and armpit hair. There are often multiple mechanisms that stop their cyclic centre from functioning correctly at work here. These include:

- stress;
- over-exercising;
- loss of fat;
- follicular malfunctioning due to low-protein diet;
- some drugs, such as antidepressants;
- multiple nutritional deficiencies, making the whole body struggle.

Regaining the weight usually results in a resumption of ovulation and periods. From then on, their diet must be balanced and they must eat adequate amounts of protein in order to nourish their system.

Hypothalamic-pituitary problems

The hypothalamus and the pituitary control all the body's major glands. Any problems in these two important areas will have

Patient story: Christina, 17 years old

Christina came to see me because she had not menstruated for three years. Her first period had occurred when she was twelve years old and they had been regular for two years. Then she lost 10 kilograms (22 pounds) in weight and not long afterwards her periods stopped. She had regained 6 kilograms (13 pounds), but her periods had not returned. She was a strict vegan (no meat, fish, eggs or dairy products), eating mostly fruit. She also went to the gym three times a week.

Christina appeared to be in good health, but had swollen ankles. Her height was 1.65 metres (5 foot 4 inches) and her weight was 45 kilograms (99 pounds), giving her a BMI of 16.5. Her blood test showed low levels of LH and FSH (indicating that her cyclic centre had switched down), low serum albumen (a blood protein) and lymphocyte (a type of white blood cell) count. These latter two are classic test results in protein deficiency. She was also deficient in iron, zinc and vitamin D.

An ultrasound scan also showed she had multicystic ovaries, not PCO. Multicystic ovaries usually indicate that the cyclic centre is suppressed, probably working only for only around half the day. I encouraged her to broaden her diet, especially to include more protein. For her this meant consuming more beans, especially soybean. I suggested she also take some supplements to treat her nutritional deficiencies. She soon began menstruating again.

significant implications for the rest of the body. Many factors can slow the function of the cyclic centre—as we have discussed, anorexia or simple weight loss, some drugs and stress, among others—and correction of these problems usually restores the cycle. However, there are a number of physical problems relating to this area of the brain that can affect this delicate control mechanism and suppress menstruation.

Kallman's syndrome

Kallman's syndrome, described in 1944, is a rare inherited condition which can affect men and women. Affected individuals are born without a hypothalamic cyclic centre and they do not mature sexually. For example, a girl will not experience breast development or spontaneous periods, and usually has no sense of smell. (The GnRH nerve cells in the cyclic center develop from the nasal area, not the brain, hence the link with lack of smell.) These girls will also be unusually tall for their age. As discussed previously, normally the pubertal surge of oestrogen fuses the growth plates in the long bones and puts a halt to growth. When there is no oestrogen, the growth plates continue to develop, and will keep growing until the affected patients are treated with oestrogen and progesterone.

This disease is often inherited in a dominant fashion—that is, half of the family members down one side are affected. We have two genes for each characteristic—one from mum and one from dad. Dominant genetic conditions produce problems with just one out of two affected genes. Some genetic disorders are recessive, meaning that both genes have to be affected to cause a problem. Kallman's syndrome usually runs in families, but it can sometimes just appear in a family without any prior cases.

To treat this condition, it is very important that the sex hormones are replaced very slowly, commencing with very small doses of oestrogen, to mimic normal puberty. This permits normal breast development. FSH or GnRH therapy usually restores normal fertility (see Chapter 6). Simple fertility drugs like clomiphene (Chapter 6) don't work in this condition.

Tumours

Tumours in the hypothalamic-pituitary area disrupt this delicate control area and usually result in an under-functioning pituitary. The exception is the pituitary adenoma, which actively secretes hormones—the commonest pituitary adenoma being prolactinoma which over-secretes prolactin. Most other tumours damage the GnRH pulse generator, resulting in low levels of LH and FSH, and so leading to low levels of sex hormones.

Sheehan's syndrome

One of the more dramatic pituitary conditions is Sheehan's syndrome, described in 1939. Severe blood loss, usually during or after childbirth, results in severe shock which may damage the pituitary. Typically, the whole pituitary shuts down. This results in a lack of pituitary drive to the thyroid, adrenals and ovaries. Early symptoms include failure to produce milk, fatigue and low blood pressure. Later symptoms include loss of armpit and pubic hair. Failure to make the diagnosis and replace the hormones may even lead to death due to lack of thyroid hormones and cortisol.

Patient story: Vicky, 17 years old
When Vicky came to see me she had not started puberty. She had had neurosurgery when she was seven for a benign pituitary tumour. She was completely cured and was on cortisone and thyroid replacement. While she had no breast or sex hair development, her blood tests revealed detectable levels of LH, FSH and prolactin. I recommended very small doses of oestrogen to induce puberty, increasing the medication six months later and so on, until she was taking a low-dose contraceptive Pill. To maximise breast development, it is important to slowly increase doses of oestrogen to mimic normal puberty. If Vicki had been started on the contraceptive Pill first, then it is doubtful that she would have experienced normal breast development—usually the breasts fail to grow to their full potential and can be small and misshapen. Later in life, she will need FSH therapy if she wants to have a baby.

Premature menopause

Menopause means 'last period'. The normal age range for the last menstrual period is anywhere between 40 and 60 years, with the average being around 51. The periods stop because there are no eggs left. Premature or early menopause may be defined as occurring when the ovaries stop working before the age of 40 years. To confirm this diagnosis, an elevated blood level of FSH of more than 40 u/L or 40 mu/mL (normal range is 2–20 u/L or 2–20 mu/mL) needs to be detected on two or three separate occasions, separated by a month each time, as there can be a lot of variation with the blood tests.

Premature menopause can run in families, or it may be part of an immune disease where the thyroid and other glands can also fail. The latter cause is associated with auto-antibodies, such as anti-ovarian and anti-thyroid antibodies, which can be detected with a blood test. Here the ovaries are attacked and gradually destroyed by the anti-ovarian antibodies. It is not clear how these antibodies come about, but there does seem to be a genetic predisposition. Sometimes early menopause may be a genetic problem—the best-known chromosomal cause of early menopause is Turner's syndrome, where one X chromosome is missing. Some treatments for cancer, such as chemotherapy or radiotherapy, may also induce an early menopause. Obviously, removing the ovaries for medical reasons will cause menopause and, as the ovaries and the uterus share some of their blood supply, even if the ovaries are left in place during a hysterectomy there is still an increased risk of early menopause, generally moving it forward by about five years.

Treatment depends on the woman's need. Early menopause increases the risk of osteoporosis and perhaps an earlier than normal increased risk of heart problems. Hormone replacement therapy may be recommended to prevent these disorders. If a younger woman has undergone premature menopause and wants to have a baby, she could consider egg donation. This is usually performed in IVF units.

Resistant ovary syndrome is a condition characterised by apparent ovarian failure while eggs are detectable in the ovaries. For some unknown reason, the remaining eggs don't respond normally to FSH stimulation. Typically, serum FSH levels vary from normal to over 40 u/L (40 mu/mL). Clinically, these women can have typical menopausal symptoms for a few months or years and then resume spontaneous ovulations again. They seem to have their best chance of spontaneous pregnancy while on hormone replacement therapy. Women who undergo a spontaneous (i.e. non-surgical) premature menopause retain a 10–15 per cent chance of resuming ovulations and conceiving while on HRT.

The cause of resistant ovary syndrome remains a mystery to medical researchers. Some of my patients have irregular periods for twenty years—others ovulate a couple of times every few years.

The main long-term health hazard for women with early menopause is osteoporosis. Calcium supplements, HRT or even the Pill can help prevent this problem. Bone density scans can be used to monitor for osteoporosis.

Patient story: Sarah, 26 years
Sarah's periods did not return after the birth of her first child. Her FSH was over 100 u/L (100 mu/mL), but her prolactin and thyroid function were normal, and her chromosomes and tissue antibodies negative. I suggested she start on HRT, and six months later she fell pregnant. After that pregnancy her periods failed to return again, but she subsequently conceived again on HRT. When her periods did not return again, she chose to go on the Pill as she didn't want any more children. Sarah clearly has resistant ovary syndrome.

Thyroid problems

The thyroid gland sits low in the front of the neck. Thyroid problems are much more common in women than in men. As thyroid hormones are essential for the normal functioning of every cell in the body, thyroid problems can certainly interfere with the menstrual cycle. Both an over-active or under-active thyroid can interfere with ovulation, and treating the thyroid problem usually restores fertility.

There are a number of diseases that cause the thyroid to become over- or under-active, including Hashimoto's disease or a 'hot nodule' in the thyroid gland (similar to a pituitary adenoma—a small lump in the gland).

A woman with under-active thyroid disease (hypothyroidism) may have heavy periods, profound tiredness and weakness, and puffiness as well as swelling and constipation. A high serum level of TSH and low free T4 confirm the diagnosis. The treatment involves giving oral T4 (thyroxine, a very long-acting hormone). When T4 treatment is started, symptoms such as sweats, tremors and palpitations can be troublesome, but soon pass as the body readapts to normal T4 levels.

Hyperthyroidism is usually due to Graves' disease or a 'hot nodule' that over-produces thyroid hormone. Graves' disease is an auto-immune condition characterised by a smooth goitre, eye manifestations and swelling over the front of the lower leg (called 'pretibial myxoedema'). A hot nodule refers to an area in the thyroid that is over-producing thyroid hormones, rather than the whole gland being over-active.

Typically, women with hyperthyroidism have a short menstrual cycle, producing frequent periods. A diagnosis is made when high levels of T4 and/or T3 and a low level of TSH are found in the bloodstream. A thyroid scan will distinguish Graves' disease from a toxic nodule.

The treatment of an over-active thyroid is usually with tablets, radio-iodine to destroy the gland, or surgery to remove most of the thyroid gland. The latter two treatments often result in hypothyroidism and the need for T4 replacement. Once normal thyroid function has been restored, it should be checked at least annually.

Patient story: Anita, 23 years old

Anita came to see me because she had irregular periods. Her ultrasound scan showed PCO, but she had also noticed fluid retention, weight gain, profound tiredness and severe constipation. I noticed that she had an obvious goitre. Blood testing showed she had a markedly under-active thyroid and strongly positive thyroid autoantibodies. Anita was prescribed thyroxine and the dose was adjusted according to thyroid function tests performed every eight weeks. When I saw Anita six months later, she was taking 150 mcg of thyroxine daily and her thyroid function tests were normal. Her periods had also returned and she felt that she was back to normal. I suggested that she have a thyroid function blood test at least annually.

Adrenal problems

There are two adrenal glands, one on each side, near the kidneys. Each adrenal is made up of an outer cortex that produces cortisone, androgens (male sex hormones) and aldosterone, a hormone that regulates salt and water. The inner part or medulla produces adrenaline. Adrenal over- or under-activity can interfere with the reproductive system.

Rarely, adrenal adenomas can cause androgen excess, and this can be misdiagnosed as PCOS. They are associated with very high levels of adrenal hormones such as DHEAS and the adenoma is usually seen on a CT or MRI scan. The adenoma is usually removed via keyhole surgery.

Congenital adrenal hyperplasia

Congenital adrenal hyperplasia (CAH) is an inherited condition where one of the adrenal enzymes is either completely or partially missing. It is usually diagnosed by performing a Synacthen (or ACTH) test. This simple test involves measuring some adrenal hormones, usually cortisol and 17-hydroxyprogesterone (17-OH-P), before and after an injection of ACTH.

Myth: All women who suffer from excess hair and irregular periods have PCOS.
Fact: Adult-type 21-hydroxylase deficiency also presents these symptoms, so it can wrongly be diagnosed as PCOS.

The most common variation of CAH is 21-hydroxylase deficiency where the enzyme 21-hydroxylase is lacking. This key enzyme is critical in the production of cortisone, and if 21-hydroxylase is not working properly, then the adrenals tend to make more androgens.

CAH is a recessive genetic disorder, so an affected individual has two abnormal genes for this enzyme. The parents are usually carriers, having one normal and one abnormal gene, and so are unaffected. However, one in four of their offspring with have a double dose of the abnormal gene and so will have the disease. The abnormal gene is common in some races such as the Celts (Irish, Northern English and Scots) and some of the Mediterranean races. Other genes regulate the expression of the 21-hydroxylase gene, so the severity of this disorder can vary from a severe foetal form to a mild late-onset variation which behaves clinically like PCOS and presents in adulthood. Babies with the severe foetal form are usually completely missing the 21-hydroxylase enzyme. The hormones that build up before the block are mostly androgens, so a female foetus will be 'masculinised', and the true sex of the baby may not be clear at birth. Also, these babies are cortisone deficient. Inside the uterus, maternal and placental cortisone maintains the foetus, but after birth the baby is cut off from this source of cortisone and will die unless given cortisone soon after birth.

The adult form of the disease is much more common than the severe foetal form. Women with late-onset CAH usually present to their doctor with excess body hair and irregular menstrual periods, and so clinically resemble PCOS sufferers. These women have a partial deficiency of 21-hydroxylase and are not usually cortisone deficient, but can have marked androgen excess. Clinically, women with the adult-type 21-hydroxylase deficiency will have the same symptoms as women with PCO syndrome—namely, menstrual irregularity and often acne and/or excess body hair.

> Women with late-onset CAH usually present to their doctor with excess body hair and irregular menstrual periods, and so clinically resemble PCOS sufferers.

The diagnosis is usually suspected by finding high bloods levels of 17-hydroxyprogesterone (the hormone that is acted upon by 21-hydroxylase). The best test to diagnose CAH is a Synacthen test. These women maintain normal adrenal cortisone production because of high ACTH levels and enlarged, overworked adrenals (caused by the increased ACTH drive). Low-dose dexamethasone (0.25–0.5 milligrams at night) suppresses ACTH levels and restores the cycle. Dexamethasone is a cortisone-like medication, but in these very low doses is safe and has few side-effects. The skin usually returns to normal after some months. As people tend to marry within their racial group, it is important to screen the male partner with a Synacthen test (see Table 5.4) to see whether he is a carrier. The test is usually normal, but if he is a carrier, then the offspring may be severely affected.

Synacthen (ACTH) normally stimulates the adrenals to release a surge of cortisol, which should rise by more than 250 nmol/L (9.1 mcg/dL) while the other adrenal hormones such as 17-hydroxy-progesterone should remain stable. People with a 21-hydroxylase deficiency may have a flat cortisol response and a significant rise in 17-hydroxyprogesterone (as shown in the table). Some will have a normal cortisol response and just the rise in 17-hydroxyprogesterone levels.

Table 5.4 Examples of Synacthen test results

	Initial	30 mins	60 mins
Normal			
Cortisol, nmol/L (mcg/dL)	270 (9.8)	590 (21.4)	640 (23.2)
17-hydroxyprogesterone, nmol/L (g/L)	1.0 (0.3)	1.5 (0.5)	2.1 (0.7)
Late-onset CAH			
Cortisol, nmol/L (mcg/dL)	220 (7.8)	380 (13.8)	350 (12.7)
17-hydroxyprogesterone, nmol/L (g/L)	45 (14.9)	150 (49.6)	250 (82.6)

Patient story: Robyn, 17 years old

As a teenager, Robyn had experienced her first period when she was twelve years old, but had had only two periods in the following five years. She then noticed worsening facial hair and acne. Her test results showed:

- total testosterone 7 nmol/L or 201.7 ng/dL (this is a high result even for PCOS—normal range less than 3 nmol/L or 86.5 ng/dL);
- 17-hydroxyprogesterone 35 nmol/L or 11.6 g/L (a very high result—normal range less than 6 nmol/L or 2 g/L);
- post-Synacthen cortisol levels of 320–720–500 nmol/L (normal);
- post-Synacthen 17-hydroxyprogesterone levels of 32–120–178 nmol/L (high).

From these results, I concluded that Robyn had the late-onset form of 21-hydroxylase deficiency. I suggested that she commence dexamethasone (0.25 milligrams at night). Her menstrual periods soon began to occur monthly, and the excess hair and acne cleared after some months.

Late-onset congential adrenal hyperplasia should be suspected when the story sounds like PCOS but the blood tests show a high level of 17-hydroxyprogesterone.

Cushing's syndrome

Cushing's syndrome, or cortisol over-production, is rare and is usually due to a pituitary adenoma, which secretes excess amounts of ACTH. This will, in turn, over-stimulate the adrenals to produce excess cortisone. Symptoms include scant and few menstrual periods, a fat tummy with relatively skinny legs, excess hair, bright red stretch marks, high blood pressure, limb weakness and a red face. The excess cortisol can also cause severe osteoporosis, resulting in easily broken bones. Cushing's syndrome can also be due to an adrenal adenoma, which is over-secreting cortisol. A simple screening test measures the 24-hour urinary-free cortisol excretion. It involves you collecting your entire urine output for 24 hours and the amount of cortisone in each collection is measured. The levels may be elevated if the person is overweight, depressed or drinks too much alcohol, but a normal result virtually excludes Cushing's syndrome. An elevated result requires further investigations.

Patient story: Sonia, 32 years old

Sonia came to see me because she had gained 30 kilograms (66 pounds) in weight over twelve months. She had also noticed bright red stretch marks on her abdomen. Also, her periods had stopped and she noticed increasing dark, coarse facial hair. When I examined Sonia, I noticed that she had a red face and was unable to get up from a squat, indicating that her thigh muscles were weak. Her blood pressure was high at 180/120 (normal is around 120/80). Her blood and urinary cortisol levels were markedly elevated, but her ACTH level was zero. MRI scans revealed a 4-centimetre (1.57-inch) right adrenal adenoma. This was removed by a laparoscopic procedure (keyhole surgery). I saw her again six months after her surgery, and found that her blood pressure was normal and she had lost most of the weight. The excess hair disappeared with a course of spironolactone (see Chapter 4).

Uterine problems

Sometimes irregular bleeding can be due to a physical problem in the uterus or pelvis. The three most common problems are fibroids, adenomyosis and endometriosis.

Fibroids are benign balls of fibrous tissue and muscle which grow on the wall of the uterus (see Figure 5.3). By age 40 years, around one in three women will have at least one fibroid. They can enlarge the uterus and are often associated with heavy menstrual bleeding and pelvic pain—although not always. Some women can develop a very large uterus, which produces pressure symptoms on the bladder causing urinary frequency, pelvic pressure, congestion, aching and fullness in the rectum, or just a heavy feeling in the pelvis. Sometimes the growing, enlarged uterus is even mistaken for a pregnancy.

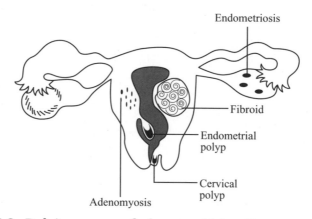

Figure 5.3 Pelvic causes of abnormal bleeding

The precise cause of fibroids remains elusive, but they appear to be driven by sex hormones, especially oestrogen. Menopause cures fibroids—they shrink dramatically in size once menstruation has stopped. Some drugs switch off the menstrual cycle by inhibiting the

GnRH cyclic centre. Nafarelin nasal spray is used twice daily, and for goserelin a monthly injection is given; both usually stop menstruation whilst the drugs are used. A six-month course of these drugs usually halves the volume of the fibroids and also produces a six-month menstrual holiday. Unfortunately, these drugs are expensive and if taken for years may result in osteoporosis (due to a prolonged lack of oestrogen). After a course of treatment, the periods usually remain lighter for some months, but often the fibroids can grow back. I often recommend these drugs to a patient in her late forties who wants to avoid surgery and is anticipating her own menopause in a couple of years. In such a case, they will often 'cure' the fibroids. A course of nafarelin will often control the fibroid problem for a few years and then her menopause will complete the shrinkage of the fibroids.

Sometimes progestins such as norethisterone (5 milligrams daily) can be used to suppress menstruation. The fibroids can also be removed surgically. If a fibroid is protruding into the uterine cavity, it can usually be removed via a small telescope called a hysteroscope. Myomectomy is an operation where large fibroids can be removed through an open operation (via an abdominal incision) or via a laparoscope (keyhole surgery). If the woman has completed her childbearing, she may choose to have the uterus removed (hysterectomy) to cure the problem. I am not aware of any clinically proven natural therapies for fibroids.

Adenomyosis is a disease where the endometrium, the lining of the uterus, grows into the muscle of the uterus, particularly the back wall, resulting in a bulky, enlarged uterus (see Figure 5.3). Ultrasound may be suggestive of adenomyosis, but often it can only be diagnosed at hysterectomy. Adenomyosis often causes a congestion-type, colicky pelvic pain, usually associated with heavy menstrual loss. The drugs described previously may help, but only hysterectomy is curative.

Endometriosis is a common and perplexing condition, characterised by the presence of tissue that resembles uterine lining—except that it is found outside the uterus, typically on the ovaries and the back of the uterus. Endometriotic implants can vary in appearance from small colourless blisters to red, inflamed lesions or dark, black 'gunpowder burns'. In severe cases, blood-filled cysts called endometriomas can enlarge the ovaries, and the pelvic structures such as the fallopian tubes, ovaries and bowel can all be caught up in dense scar tissue.

The cause of endometriosis is still the subject of much speculation, but there are two main theories: implantation and transformation. Bleeding out the fallopian tubes at the time of menstruation is common and so endometrial cells can be carried into the pelvis where they may implant. Why these cells implant and grow in some and not others is unknown. The abdominal cavity is lined by a smooth layer called the peritoneum that permits the bowel and other contents to slide over each other. The transformation theory suggests that some of the peritoneum that lines the pelvis is converted into cells that resemble the endometrium. Both theories require other factors to permit implantation or transformation.

The severity of the endometriosis does not necessarily correlate with the symptoms. Some women have no symptoms, and endometriosis may be found incidentally during an elective procedure such as tubal sterilisation. Others have a few spots of endometriosis and yet have crippling pain. However, the main symptoms include pelvic pain—particularly with menstruation or sexual intercourse—irregular uterine bleeding and sometimes trouble conceiving. The pain is usually associated with menstrual periods, but may start before menstruation and continue after the cessation of menses. Nodules of endometriosis at the back of the uterus can be tender and bumped during sexual intercourse, eliciting pain (see Figure 5.4). Most of the nerve supply to the uterus enters via the ligaments at the back of the uterus, so endometriosis at this site can be particularly painful. The classic menstrual symptom of endometriosis is premenstrual spotting, which can be quite troublesome and usually resolves with successful therapy. Endometriosis may be found at diagnostic laparoscopy for an infertility work-up. It is important that a complete evaluation be performed on a sub-fertile couple, even if endometriosis is found, as combined problems are not uncommon.

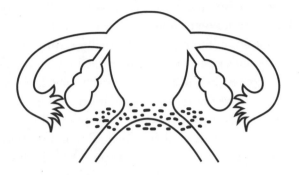

Figure 5.4 Endometriosis

The medical treatment of endometriosis may be divided into short- or long-term therapy. Short-term therapy may be given for one to three months as a prelude to surgery, or for six months as a course of therapy. A GnRH agonist (nafarelin or goserelin) or danazol is probably the best method of treatment in this regard because these have a relatively rapid effect, but their side-effects preclude their long-term use. Danazol may have male hormone-like side-effects such as weight gain, oily skin, hirsutism and acne. These may be minimised by using 400 milligrams rather than the original 800 milligram dosage, and by encouraging the woman to exercise. GnRH agonists have a very low rate of side-effects from the drug itself but, because they effectively switch off the ovaries, GnRH agonists produce a low-oestrogen state so that symptoms such as hot flushes and vaginal dryness can be a problem. In overseas trials, long-term (more than six months) use of GnRH agonists has been combined with low dose HRT, especially tibolone, to avoid these problems and prevent bone loss. Laparoscopic surgery is increasingly being used to treat endometriosis, so the main indication for drug therapy is as a long-term treatment for the endometriosis and contraception, preserving the pelvis until pregnancy is desired. In this respect, progestins are in their own class.

Progestins have a long history of use in contraceptives

(e.g. Depot-Provera, Implanon, progesterone-only Pills, combined contraceptive Pills). Medroxyprogesterone acetate (MPA) (30 milligrams) or norethisterone (5 milligrams daily) usually results in a cessation of menstruation by the second or third month and is an effective contraceptive. Some women like to have a monthly bleed, so they can take these drugs for 21 days out of 28. Progestins may not be contraceptive if taken cyclically. About 10 per cent of women will notice PMT-type side-effects, including pelvic bloatedness, irritability, headaches and depression. Probably the best-tolerated progestin is dydrogesterone, but it is the only one that does not inhibit ovulation and so is probably not a contraceptive. Cyproterone acetate is also an alternative and has been used with Diane-35 as a treatment for endometriosis (25 milligrams of CPA is taken with the active Diane Pills). CPA and Diane are very useful treatments for excess hair and acne. Some women obtain good pain relief by using a fixed dose (meaning the dose of hormones is the same in each active Pill) contraceptive Pill (e.g. Microgynon 30 or Marvelon) twelve weeks on and one week off. These long-cycle contraceptive Pill regimens can be a very simple and safe solution, although sometimes the oestrogen component seems to stimulate endometriosis. Breakthrough bleeding—that is, bleeding whilst on active tablets—can be a problem, however. If significant bleeding occurs earlier than twelve weeks, then stopping active Pills for seven days usually resolves the problem.

Patient story: Louise, 47 years old
Louise consulted her GP because her periods were very heavy. She was found to be anaemic and iron deficient. An ultrasound scan confirmed an enlarged fibroid uterus—there were lots of small fibroids visible, all under 1 centimetre (0.39 inches) in diameter, but there was one 5 centimetre (1.97 inch) fibroid protruding into the cavity of the uterus. The lining of the uterus was noted to be thin. Louise wanted to know her treatment options. I suggested the following options to her:

- Put up with it. Iron tablets may correct the anaemia and menopause will cure the fibroids—if menopause happens soon. Unfortunately, there is no way of predicting when menopause will occur.
- Norethisterone (5 milligrams daily) to try to suppress menstruation. About one in eight women develop PMT-type side-effects such as irritability and bloatedness.
- Nafarelin nasal spray switches off the cyclic centre and so turns off menstruation. A six-month course of nafarelin nasal spray will usually shrink the fibroids, but they may grow back again after the course is finished. In Australia the drug costs about A$100 per month, but most private health funds will refund some of that. During the treatment, some women notice menopausal-type hot flushes, but they are usually mild. If nafarelin is taken for years, then the prolonged lack of oestrogen may result in osteoporosis. However, it can be a very useful drug in this setting, where menopause is anticipated within a couple of years.
- The main 5-centimetre (1.97 inch) fibroid can be removed via an hysteroscope, and at the same time the lining of the uterus can be burned and removed (an endometrial ablation) to make the periods lighter. The effects of this treatment usually last for about five years.
- Hysterectomy or removal of the uterus is the definitive treatment. The operation can often be performed laparoscopically, so the hospital stay is usually only a couple of days.

What can I do to control menstrual problems?

Many women who are not menstruating do not want to become pregnant immediately; however, they need some treatment before and between pregnancies. Either their ovaries are inactive and they are not producing sex hormones (therefore putting them at risk of osteoporosis) or they are producing oestrogen without progesterone to protect the lining of the uterus, consequently putting them at increased risk of cancer of the uterus. Women with PCOS may also be at increased risk of uterine cancer, but not osteoporosis. Blood measurement of oestradiol is of no value in this situation, as it will not detect other oestrogens, such as oestrone and oestriol, which may be elevated in different hormonal conditions.

A simple way in which your doctor can distinguish which of these two groups you belong to is to prescribe 10 milligrams of a synthetic progestin, such as MPA, daily for five days. Any bleeding that ensues within seven days of taking the progestin (including brown discharge) indicates that some oestrogen activity is present, as it has stimulated the endometrium. Put another way, progestins will only make you bleed if oestrogenised endometrium is present. If you are not ovulating, but have some oestrogen activity present, then you will require endometrial protection. If left untreated there may be an increased risk of endometrial cancer (see Chapter 8) as well as the occasional very heavy period when the thick oestrogen-induced uterine lining is lost. A lack of bleeding after a progestin challenge suggests a low oestrogen state, so the main hazard is an increased risk of developing osteoporosis. Quite reasonably, some women will not want to take a medical treatment unless absolutely necessary. Having a bone density scan every year or two can monitor the bone mass of those with a low oestrogen condition. If the bone density starts to decline, then oestrogen treatment should be instituted.

The combined Pill remains a good treatment for both groups of women, as it will protect both the bones and the uterine lining. If contraception is not required, then a progestin can be taken for twelve to fourteen days every month or two to induce menstrual bleeding. This will protect the uterus from malignant change and prevent the buildup of a thick endometrium. If a low-oestrogen state is diagnosed, then HRT or an OCP can be used. Young women with oestrogen deficiency generally require more oestrogen than older menopausal women. However, it is important to remember that hormone replacement therapy is *not* a contraceptive.

Short-term therapies to control heavy periods

There are two simple medical approaches to stopping a heavy period. The first involves starting a contraceptive Pill. In general, the stronger the Pill, the faster the bleeding will be controlled. Microgynon 20 may take two to three months to control very heavy periods, whereas Microgynon 50 might control the problem from the first tablet. I usually suggest that an ultrasound scan be performed to check the thickness of the endometrium and to see whether there are any physical uterine problems present, such as fibroids.

Patient story: Jennifer, 37 years old
Jennifer was known to have PCOS and came to see me because she had been bleeding for two weeks. I could not find any physical problems when I examined her. Jennifer's blood tests and scan were normal. I suggested that she take Microgynon 50 for four months. When I saw her again four months later, her periods were regular and light so I suggested she swap to Microgynon 30.

The second medical approach to a heavy, persistent period is a moderate dosage of a progestin, such as norethisterone. The dosage varies according to the severity of the problem, but it would be usual for me to suggest a woman in this situation take one or two tablets (each containing 5 milligrams of norethisterone) three to four times a day initially, to control the bleeding problem, then take a smaller dosage for at least three to four weeks to shrink the lining of the uterus. When the drug is stopped, a light period usually follows. It is a very safe method, but these doses can cause some bloatedness, mood swings and irritability.

Patient story: Donna, aged 32 years
Donna came to see me after having spent the night in the local casualty department. She was having a heavy period for two weeks. The casualty doctor had ordered a blood count, a pregnancy test and an ultrasound scan. All these tests were normal, except that the scan had shown that the lining of her uterus was thick and that she had PCO. She had been started on two tablets of norethisterone three times daily. Now, three days later, she had stopped bleeding. I suggested that she continue on that dose for about seven days, then reduce the dose to one three times a day and continue on that for another three weeks and then have a week off. When I saw her again, during the week off the norethisterone, she was having a light period.

Long-term therapies to control heavy periods

Twenty or more years ago, removal of the uterus (a hysterectomy) was the main long-term method for controlling heavy periods. This was usually performed through a large cut on the abdomen, so the woman had to spend one to two weeks in hospital to recover, and then needed another month or two off work. In the past ten years, the situation has radically changed, so much so that I personally no longer perform hysterectomies. The best treatment will vary according to the individual's wishes and the cause of the heavy periods. The following are some of the long-term options to control heavy periods.

Anti-inflammatory tablets
Anti-inflammatory tablets, such as mefenamic acid or naproxen, can be effective not just for period pain, but also to reduce menstrual flow, if started immediately at the onset of a period and taken in full dosage for four to five days. Many women take a couple of capsules of these as needed for period pain, but to reduce menstrual flow they need to be taken continually during the period.

The contraceptive Pill

It is well known that the contraceptive Pill substantially reduces menstrual blood flow, but some women continue to have heavy periods even while they are on the Pill. Another useful strategy is to take a fixed-dose pill, such as Microgynon 30, Marvelon or Yasmin, continually. Clinical trials have shown that most women can take these for up to twelve weeks without too much irregular bleeding. My usual advice is to take them until significant bleeding occurs and then have a week off before restarting. A day or two of spotting can be ignored, but persistent spotting or bleeding indicates that the week-off therapy should be followed. If the Pill is continued, then the bleeding usually worsens.

The bleeding occurs because the endometrium becomes very thin, exposing underlying blood vessels, which then bleed. The week off allows the uterine lining to regenerate. As time goes by, the menstrual control gets better and better. Many of my patients have only two to three periods a year. This is safe, and is a more effective contraceptive than the usual 'three weeks on/one week off' regimen. If a special event is coming up, such as a holiday or an exam, then the Pills can be deliberately stopped two to three weeks before the event to bring on a period.

Progestins

Another approach is to take a moderate dose of a progestin, either continuously or for three weeks on and one week off. Depo-Provera is a three-month injection of MPA that stops menstruation in around 85 per cent of women. Side-effects include bloatedness, mood swings and irregular bleeding. Using tablets of progestin such as MPA (20 to 30 milligrams) or norethisterone (5 milligrams) daily can achieve the same effect.

Transexamic acid

Transexamic acid is a treatment that helps stop bleeding blood vessels. It is very effective for heavy periods, particularly when the uterus is apparently normal (i.e. no fibroids or adenomyosis). Clinical trials have shown that it reduces menstrual blood loss even more effectively than the Pill. Most of the uterine lining is lost on day one of the menstrual period, after which the blood lost is mostly from small, torn blood vessels. Transexamic acid helps to plug these bleeding vessels. The usual starting dose is 1 gram three times a day, from days one to five of menstruation. Doses of up to 1.5 grams four times a day have been used. Normally it is extremely well tolerated, with few side-effects. The main side-effect is nausea, which is uncommon and usually settles with a dosage reduction and taking the medication with food.

The Mirena device

The Mirena device is a novel treatment for heavy periods. This is a progestin-containing intrauterine device (IUD), which delivers levonorgestrel (LG) topically to the endometrium. Blood levels of the LG are extremely low (over a 100 times lower than the mini-Pill), so progestin side-effects are very uncommon. Many women have irregular light spotting for up to three months after insertion, but after that have monthly, very light menstrual bleeding. The effect of the device lasts at least five years and, because it contains progestin, cervical mucus is thickened, lowering the risk of pelvic infection. The risk of endometrial cancer is also reduced. The device can also be removed easily, making it an ideal option for women with very heavy periods who haven't yet completed their family. I have found the Mirena device an excellent option for women with complex medical problems who have heavy periods and/or who need contraception. I have fitted the device to women who have had breast cancer, kidney or liver failure or clots in the lung. The device offers excellent menstrual control, reversible contraception and minimal side-effects because hardly any of the active hormone actually gets into the bloodstream.

Conservative surgery

For the minority of women with heavy periods who need surgery, keyhole surgery has greatly improved the options. Endoscopic surgery involves the use of small telescopes to perform the operation through small keyhole incisions. Endometrial ablation involves burning the lining of the uterus. A variety of techniques can be used, including burning using an electrical current, laser, microwaves or a balloon-filled hot water system. Results seem similar to those obtained with the Mirena device. Some will be advised to have a hysterectomy, especially if a malignant or pre-malignant disease is present, or if the uterus is greatly enlarged—usually due to fibroids (muscular growths in the wall of the uterus).

Hysterectomy

If a decision has been made to have a hysterectomy, then it is vital that careful consideration be given to whether it is performed vaginally or through a cut on the abdomen. Vaginal hysterectomy is usually performed if there is some degree of prolapse—that is, if the uterus is tending to drop down and if the uterus is small enough. Vaginal hysterectomy is often performed as part of a vaginal repair operation; otherwise, the operation is performed through a low transverse incision ('bikini cut'). Vaginal hysterectomy is associated with less post-operative discomfort than the abdominal operation. However, the discomfort of the abdominal operation can be minimised if the wound is infiltrated with long-acting local anaesthetic and by the judicious use of a narcotic drip and non-steroidal anti-inflammatories. There is also increasing interest in laparoscopic-assisted vaginal hysterectomy (LAVH). This procedure involves keyhole surgery—dissecting the uterus 'from above' and then removing the uterus vaginally. Another novel laparoscopic approach involves removing just the top part of the uterus and leaving the cervix (laparoscopic subtotal hysterectomy). The major blood supply to the uterus and the bladder and ureters (the tubes that join the bladder to the kidneys) is down near the cervix, so a subtotal hysterectomy is safer and quicker than the total hysterectomy. However, as the cervix remains with the subtotal-type operation, pap smears need to continue after the operation. Over the last decade laparoscopic surgery has emerged as a sub-specialty and now I have colleagues who basically only perform this type of surgery. I have found that my patients who have had laparoscopic surgery recover much more quickly than those who've had an abdominal hysterectomy.

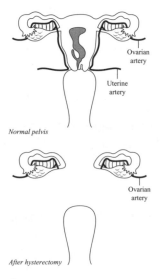

Figure 5.5 Hysterectomy

Summary

Menstrual irregularity is common, and polycystic ovaries are often found during the investigation of this condition. However, the presence of PCO does not necessarily mean it is the cause of the problem. About 25 per cent of reproductive-aged women have scan evidence of PCO, so it is possible to have PCO and another cause of menstrual irregularity. However, the presence of excess body hair would strongly suggest that PCOS is the cause. Rarely, adrenal conditions such as CAH can mimic PCOS. Menstrual problems can be due to physical conditions in the uterus such as fibroids, adenomyosis and endometriosis.

In the end, all women with menstrual irregularity should have a blood test to measure their hormone profile and to identify the cause. An ultrasound scan not only gives information about the ovaries, but also detects many uterine problems. Most women with heavy periods can be offered one or more suitable medical options. For those who choose, or need to have, surgery, keyhole surgery offers considerable advantages over the older abdominal approach.

Frequently asked questions

I've been having a very heavy period for ten days now. Can I take something to stop it?

Yes. Norethisterone tablets taken three times a day usually help a lot. The norethisterone should be taken for about four weeks, then stopped. Usually a light withdrawal period results. It might be worth doing some tests to investigate the bleeding. These might include an ultrasound scan, a blood count and some hormone levels.

I have PCOS and my periods have always been irregular, coming about twice a year. Is there any chance that my periods will regulate themselves?

Yes. Around 20–25 per cent of women with PCOS will spontaneously have regular periods for a time. Often, a low-GI, low-fat diet (see Chapter 7) and exercise will encourage a natural, regular cycle.

6
Producing results:
Fertility issues

Fertility is a big issue for most women. Up to around 50 years ago, many women were married at a young age—eighteen to twenty years—conceived immediately and had between eight and twelve children over their lifetime. There were few good contraceptive choices. Today, most women are waiting until they are in their thirties to try for a baby. It is well known that female fertility declines with age—for two main reasons. First, as women age, so do their eggs. If you are 30 years old, then your eggs are about 31 years old. Second, as you age, there is an increased risk of developing a problem (such as appendicitis, endometriosis, a pelvic infection) that might impair fertility. Some men find that their sperm count falls with increasing age. So infertility specialists like myself are seeing more and more women having trouble conceiving.

However, as we have already discussed, many women with PCO are incorrectly told that they are infertile. Some young women think this means that they can have unprotected sex—then they find themselves unexpectedly pregnant. Many of my patients with PCOS seem to have no trouble conceiving either. However, some do need help to get pregnant, while others need contraception. We will examine both sides of the fertility conundrum now.

Am I infertile?

Dr Eva Dahlgren and her research team have been studying a group of Swedish women who had PCOS diagnosed in the 1950s and 1960s (Dahlgren et al., 1992). They found that about 20 per cent of the participants had regular periods at some stage of their life; for some, this was following a pregnancy. This is consistent with my experience. About ten years ago, one of my research team followed up a group of my patients with PCOS who hadn't been to see me for at least five years. We found that 25 per cent were now having regular periods. This would suggest that in some cases menstrual irregularities come and go.

Dr Dahlgren also found that of the women who wanted to be pregnant, 76 per cent had at least one baby. Our 'thousand cases of PCOS' study gave similar results. There were 790 pregnancies among the 1019 women with PCOS before the study. Only 144 (14 per cent) presented with infertility. After fully investigating these women and their partners, we found that only eight had 'unexplained infertility' (Table 6.1). This was only 5.6 per cent of the group. Most studies have shown that between 10 and 20 per cent of infertile couples are 'unexplained'. Once a 'problem' is found (such as PCOS) there is a natural tendency to blame it for everything.

A British study (Hassan and Killick, 2003) found that women with PCO and no symptoms were just as fertile as those with normal ovaries. If you have polycystic ovaries and regular periods, it is very unlikely that you will have trouble getting pregnant. Symptoms of ovulation include mid-cycle pelvic pain, premenstrual irritability, bloatedness and breast soreness—these aren't very nice but indicate that you probably are having regular ovulations. As we shall discuss later, ovulation can be tracked with temperature charts and ovulation detection kits.

If you have polycystic ovaries and regular periods, it is very unlikely that you will have trouble getting pregnant.

Table 6.1 Infertility causes of 144 women with PCOS

Cause of infertility	Number of cases (per cent)
Blocked tubes	40 (28)
Sperm problems	35 (24)
Cervical problems	4 (3)
Infrequent ovulations alone	47 (33)
Endometriosis	39 (27)
Fibroids	6 (4)
Unexplained	8 (6)

Note: These figures are very similar to other series. When there is a fertility difficulty, about a third of the time the problem lies with the women, a third of the time with the male partner, and a third of the time with both. Some had more than one cause for their infertility.

In my experience, most women with PCOS and even irregular periods can conceive. I have seen many women with PCOS who have one or two periods a year and who have several children, never having taken fertility drugs. Some couples are very fertile and only need one or two ovulations to conceive. Those having problems usually respond well to fertility drugs.

On the other hand, many women with PCO or PCOS need to use contraception if they are sexually active and don't want to conceive. Some with PCOS may have special contraceptive requirements.

Do I need contraception?

Many women with PCOS believe they are infertile. Quite reasonably, most interpret this in two ways. First, they might assume they cannot have children—ever. In fact, many of the women I have seen with PCOS who wanted children have had them without any help from doctors. However, some do need help to conceive. Second, they might think they don't need contraception, and unexpectedly become pregnant. In my 'thousand cases of PCOS' study, there were 790 pregnancies, of which 122 were terminated. Most of the women told me they thought they couldn't have children, so they were very surprised to find out that they were pregnant. Therefore, contraception is important for women with PCOS.

Most of the time, the contraception choices for women with PCOS are similar to those facing other women. However, there may be some special circumstances to consider for those with PCOS. The range of choices includes:

- barriers, such as condoms and diaphragms;
- intrauterine devices;
- the contraceptive Pill;
- injectible contraceptives;
- sterilisation;
- natural family planning.

Barrier contraceptives

The ancient Egyptians used penile sheaths or condoms at least 3000 years ago. Originally they were made of animal intestines, then later from materials such as linen or silk, and most recently from rubber or plastic. A diaphragm is a round piece of plastic or rubber that is designed to cover the cervix and prevent sperm from entering the uterus. Used properly, both condoms and diaphragms have around a 90 per cent success rate per year. This means that if 100 couples are using a diaphragm or condoms for contraception, then ten couples per year will have an unexpected pregnancy. This rate can be improved by using a spermicidal cream with the contraceptive barrier. For example, spermicidal cream can be placed high in the vagina before sex begins, in case the condom breaks. Similarly, spermicidal cream can be placed around the rim and in the centre of the diaphragm. Recently a 'female condom' has become available. This is a plastic sheath that is placed at the entrance of the vagina at the commencement of vaginal sex. Great care should be taken when removing either a male or female condom to avoid spilling semen into the vagina.

Barrier methods of contraception are safe, simple and offer some protection against sexually transmitted diseases. Many of my patients with PCOS are happy to use these contraceptive methods.

Intrauterine devices

The concept of an intrauterine device (IUD) has been around for many years. However, the modern IUD became available in the 1960s when copper wire was added to the device, which allowed it to be made much smaller than before. One device—the Dalkon shield—caused a lot of problems with pelvic infection, leading to chronic pelvic pain and infertility. The Dalkon shield had a number of design faults, including a multifilament string and a shape that seemed to allow vaginal germs access into the uterine cavity. Modern copper/silver-containing IUDs appear to have only a very small increased risk of infection. In some countries such as China, IUDs remain a very popular contraceptive method because they are cheap, reliable and long-acting.

The newest IUD is the Mirena device, which is an excellent option for those with PCOS as it offers excellent reversible contraception, menstrual lightening and protection against uterine cancer. Many women have irregular light spotting for up to three months after insertion, but after that they have monthly very light menstrual bleeding—often just one to two days of light brown staining. The device is effective for at least five years and, because it contains progestin, cervical mucus is thickened, lowering the risk of pelvic infection. The risk of premalignant and cancerous changes of the uterine lining are also reduced. The device can also be easily removed (there's a soft string attached to it), making it an excellent option if you have very heavy periods but haven't yet completed your family.

The contraceptive Pill (the Pill)

The Pill was introduced over 40 years ago and no other medication has been more extensively investigated. There are two types of contraceptive Pills—combined Pills containing the two female hormones, oestrogen and progestin, and progestin-only pills. For most women, a combined Pill is the best and safest form of reversible contraception. Also, many women with PCOS who have acne find that combined Pills usually improve their skin problem substantially and those with excess hair find that the Pill usually, at the very least, stops their hair problem from getting worse and it may even improve it slightly.

Combined contraceptive Pills contain ethinyl oestradiol as the oestrogen and, until recently, either norethisterone or levonorgestrel as the progestin. They are now available with the antiandrogenic (male-hormone blocking) progestin cyproterone (e.g. Diane-35) or the new third-generation progestins, desogestrel (Marvelon) or gestodene (Femoden-ED, Triodcn-ED, Minulet, Tri-Minulet). The Pill has a number of anti-fertility actions. These include inhibiting the release of the egg, thickening cervical mucus to prevent sperm penetration into the uterus and an effect on the lining of the uterus.

The newer Pills contain novel progestins, which have low rates of side-effects. Some, such as Diane-35, are very useful for treating some excess hair or acne. Marvelon, Yasmin and Microgynon 20 can also be useful for female acne. Yasmin is the newest contraceptive Pill on the market. It contains drospirenone, a new category of progestin—one that closely resembles the natural hormone, progesterone. The oestrogen component, ethinyl oestradiol, tends to cause fluid retention; however, drospirenone counteracts this fluid retention. It is probably equivalent to taking 25 milligrams of spironolactone (see

Chapter 4). In clinical trials, Yasmin users on average lost half a kilogram (1 pound) in weight compared with those using the older style Pills, who generally gained a little weight. Unlike older progestins, which can cause PMT-like side-effects, Yasmin usually improves PMT. If you have taken older Pills and become moody or depressed, then Yasmin is probably worth trying. Yasmin also improves the lipid profile in the blood by raising the 'good' cholesterol fraction, HDL-cholesterol. Lastly, like Diane-35, Yasmin has an anti-androgen effect on skin, making it a useful treatment for excess hair and acne. Yasmin is therefore an excellent contraceptive Pill for those with PCOS.

Side-effects of the Pill

Modern contraceptive Pills have far fewer side-effects than the original Pill, but side-effects can still occur. Some women should probably avoid taking the Pill altogether, including those suffering from:

- breast cancer;
- uterine cancer;
- undiagnosed vaginal bleeding;
- active liver disease;
- severe systemic lupus erythematosus;
- porphyria;
- a history of clots in the leg or chest;
- heart disease;
- stroke.

The Pill is also unsuitable for heavy smokers over 40 years of age who will not quit, and it may aggravate gallstones in some vulnerable women.

Some women avoid the Pill because they are very concerned about the risk of breast cancer, heart disease, strokes and clots. If you are healthy and do not smoke, then you can take the Pill up to the age of 50 without any great risks. Most studies show no increased risk of breast cancer, or an increased risk so low it is difficult to measure—perhaps one to two extra cases per 100 000 users. (Bear in mind that the risk of death on the roads is between one and twenty per 10 000 per year and that two alcoholic drinks per day increases the risk of breast cancer more than whether or not you take the Pill.) Smokers do have a substantially increased risk of heart disease, and if a smoker is over the age of 40 then the combined contraceptive Pill does seem to be a further factor. Of course, if the smoker gives up the cigarettes, the risk will be significantly reduced.

For the vast majority of women, the Pill does not increase their risk of stroke, but there are some who need to be a bit wary. These include:

- a small number who develop high blood pressure while taking the Pill;
- some severe migraine sufferers;
- women who have had a stroke;
- women with a clotting problem (e.g. Leiden Factor V mutation).

High blood pressure usually takes at least three months to develop and can be quite mild. Stopping the Pill usually normalises the blood pressure within three to four months. As a precaution, always get the doctor or nurse to check your blood pressure before renewing your prescription.

Blood clots are a potentially very serious condition, but again the increased risk needs to be put into perspective. There is an increased risk of an extra four cases (a jump from twelve to sixteen per 100 000 per year) for a young person taking the Pill. Compared with the road toll statistics, this risk would seem to be minimal. This small extra risk seems to relate to some having rare clotting disorders, the commonest type being Leiden Factor V mutation. So if you have a family or personal history of clotting, make sure you tell your doctor. Interestingly, the risk of a deep vein thrombosis causing a clot during pregnancy is around 60 per 100 000 women per year. In other words, pregnancy is a much greater risk factor for clots than taking the oral contraceptive Pill.

Health benefits of contraceptive Pills

There are many long-term benefits from taking the contraceptive Pill. These are:

- safe and reversible prevention of pregnancy;
- fewer tubal pregnancies;
- reduced acne;
- less excess body hair;
- reduced risk of cancer of the ovary;
- reduced risk of cancer of the uterus;
- 50 per cent less pelvic infection;
- less likelihood of endometriosis;
- 50–80 per cent fewer ovarian cysts;
- predictable, lighter and less painful periods;
- less anaemia (because the menstrual periods are lighter);
- less premenstrual tension and period pain;
- no menopausal symptoms while taking it;
- maintenance of bone mass;
- fewer benign breast lumps;
- possibly less thyroid disease and rheumatoid arthritis.

Myth: The contraceptive Pill causes infertility.
Fact: The Pill is a safe way to prevent pregnancy and its effects are reversible for women during their reproductive years.

The contraceptive Pill does not cause infertility. Around one in 100 will come off the Pill, not have a period for six months and not be pregnant. Often, when these cases are investigated, a pre-existing problem—usually PCOS—will be found. Contraceptive Pills protect against a number of conditions that can cause infertility—it lowers the risk of pelvic infections, ovarian cysts and endometriosis.

If you have raised levels of triglycerides (see Chapter 7), then the oestrogen portion of the Pill can raise them even further.

Cancer of the uterus and ovary are increasingly common as women age, so the protective effect of the Pill on these common cancers is of more relevance to those over 40 years of age. Those with PCOS are also probably at slightly increased risk of uterine cancer, so this protective effect of the Pill is of particular benefit.

For those with PCOS, the Pill can very useful. Periods are regulated, uterine cancer is prevented and skin problems such as hirsutism and acne are usually improved. However, those with insulin resistance need to be a little careful. If you have raised levels of triglycerides (see Chapter 7), then the oestrogen portion of the Pill can raise them even further. It is a good idea to check that the triglyceride levels are normal before commencing the Pill. It may also be prudent to recheck blood fat levels (cholesterol and triglycerides) after using the Pill for two to three months.

Injectible contraception

The most well known of the injectible contraceptions is Implanon. It is a single, 'match-stick-sized' rod (2 millimetres by 4 centimetres or 0.08 by 1.57 inches) that slowly releases a progestin called etonogestrel, so Implanon is a progestin-only contraceptive. The rod is inserted under local anaesthetic just under the skin of the upper arm. It can be removed under a local as well. Generally the menstrual periods are much lighter and less painful; however, sometimes irregular spotting can occur. Around 10 per cent of women using this method can have side-effects such as headaches, acne or breast pain. PMS-type side-effects occur in only 5 per cent of women. The pregnancy rate is very low. When the device is removed, fertility returns immediately with no delay. The situations where Implanon may be useful include when a woman:

- suffers from nausea or breast soreness with oral therapies;
- has a history of bowel or stomach complaints;
- forgets to take the oral contraceptive Pill regularly.

Implanon is a useful option for some women with PCO or PCOS. Oestrogen tends to raise blood triglycerides and, as some women with insulin resistance have quite high blood triglyceride levels, a combined Pill could aggravate the problem. Usually Implanon does not have this effect.

Sterilisation

Many women in their mid- to late thirties suffer from increased menstrual problems such as breast pain and PMT. These can be controlled with the combined contraceptive Pill, but the burden of continuing to take the Pill may lead some women to investigate the option of sterilisation. Sterilisation includes tubal ligation or, in extreme cases, a hysterectomy for women and a vasectomy for men. Tubal ligation involves blocking the fallopian tube using endoscopic surgery, which involves the use of small telescopes to perform the operation through small 'keyhole' incisions in the navel and pubic areas.

There are some new keyhole operations that can be performed from below. Professor Thierry Vancaille, from the Royal Hospital for Women in Sydney, has invented a sterilisation system called Adiana. The procedure can be done in about ten minutes under a local anaesthetic. A hysteroscope is used to inspect the cavity of the uterus, then a tiny sponge is inserted into the hole leading to the fallopian tube (on each side). The sponge blocks the tube and so prevents pregnancy. Eventually the sponge blends into the normal tissue, but the tube remains blocked.

A hysterectomy involves the removal of the uterus and/or the cervix, but not the fallopian tubes or ovaries. A vasectomy involves blocking the vas deferens, the long duct along which sperm cells travel, by surgical means.

If you and your partner are considering sterilisation and you have been taking the Pill up until now, it may be prudent to trial not being on the Pill, using a barrier method instead, for three to four months before the operation. This will enable you to find out what your cycle will be like once you are off the Pill, as after sterilisation your ovaries will still be working as usual. Many women come off the Pill after surgery only to find that life is miserable because of the hormonal effects.

One reasonable approach if you are healthy and a non-smoker is to stay on the Pill until you are 50 years old, then stop to have your FSH levels measured. If the levels are high (more than 40 u/L or 40 mu/mL), you could consider using HRT or perhaps a natural therapy (e.g. black cohosh extract or a diet high in phytoestrogens) if hot flushes are a problem. Another approach would be to simply stop taking the Pill at 50 and see what happens.

Sterilisation is a convenient option for some with PCOS. However, if your periods are irregular and heavy, then a Mirena device or a contraceptive Pill might be better, as these two offer reversible contraception and menstrual control.

Natural family planning

Many practising Catholics use natural family planning. This involves careful study of the menstrual cycle, often involving temperature charts and study of cervical mucus. Fertile cervical mucus is a bit like egg white and lasts between three and eight days. Sex is avoided around the fertile time. There are a number of good books and websites dealing with this method, including www.billings-centre.ab.ca, but the best results are obtained by attending classes on natural family planning. If you have PCOS and only a couple of periods per year, then this method may be less reliable.

But what if I want to have a baby?

As I have already discussed, many women with PCOS will have no trouble conceiving. Understandably, these women want to maximise their chances of conceiving as quickly as possible after coming off their contraception. Some women, however, will fail to ovulate, and they will need some medical assistance. In this section I shall talk about both scenarios.

In general, it is a good idea to see your doctor about three to four months prior to coming off the Pill, to make sure your pap smear test is up to date and to have a pre-pregnancy blood test. For example, if your immunity to rubella (German measles) has worn off, it is better to find out before you are pregnant so that you can be immunised. A blood count will check for anaemia. A blood group and antibody screen is important as well, as some women have antibodies against a particular blood group and these antibodies might attack the baby's red blood cells. At this time, if you haven't already done so, you should also commence taking a folate supplement (containing at least 400 micrograms of folate [folic acid]). Deficiency of this B-group vitamin is associated with an increased risk of spina bifida in the baby.

Am I ovulating?

If you are having regular periods every 21–35 days, it is very likely that you are ovulating. Ovulation is often, but not always, associated with various symptoms. Some have pelvic pain around the time of ovulation and may notice an increase in the 'egg-white' type mucus in the days leading up to ovulation. The two weeks following ovulation are often associated with some symptoms of PMT. These may include mood changes, breast soreness, abdominal bloatedness and headaches. Day one period pain is also often associated with a preceding ovulation.

In contrast, most women who fail to ovulate don't menstruate or, if they do, do not have PMT symptoms, ovulation pain or day one period pain. In my experience, most of those with PCOS do ovulate—they just do so infrequently.

> In my experience, most of those with PCOS do ovulate—they just do so infrequently.

Temperature charts to detect ovulation
If a test of ovulation is required, usually the simplest one is a basal body temperature chart (BBTc). I usually recommend that an oral temperature is taken first thing in the morning, before getting out of bed. Charts should be kept from day one of the cycle to the commencement of the next period, when a new chart is commenced. Daily temperatures are plotted on to graph paper. You should expect some daily variation. With an ovulatory chart, temperature dips at ovulation, then rises about ½–1 degree Celsius (1–2 degrees Fahrenheit) and stays up for ten to fourteen days. If pregnancy does not occur, the temperature falls and a period ensues between one and three days later. If pregnancy occurs, the temperature remains up.

You can't use BBTc to time sex. By the time your temperature has gone up, you have already ovulated; however, basal body temperature is a very useful starting point to confirm ovulation and plan other tests.

Patient story: Amanda, 29 years old
Amanda's periods come every 35 days. She notices some mild moodiness and breast soreness for the week before her periods. Amanda has some crampy period pain on days 1 and 2 of her periods. Her BBTc is shown in Figure 6.1.

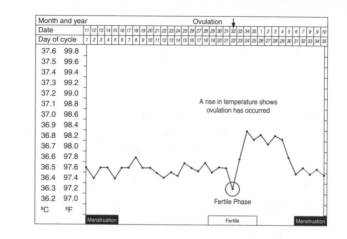

Figure 6.1 Basal body temperature chart (BBTc)

Amanda has probably ovulated on day 22 of this cycle. Notice how her temperature 'dipped' before it went up.

Ovulation detection kits

There are several ovulation detection kits available today. In my opinion, the best ones are the urinary LH-detection kits. Having used a BBTc for a couple of cycles and established when you probably ovulate, these kits can nail down the day to within 24 hours. LH-detection kits identify the LH-surge, the hormone event that triggers ovulation and that usually occurs 24–36 hours prior to ovulation. They work a bit like a pregnancy test, except that they pick up LH rather than the pregnancy hormone, HCG. The LH-detection kits typically have five non-reusable sticks in a box. Using Amanda (see patient story above) as an example, she should start testing her urine (first sample of the day) from day 17–18 of her cycle. Once the test stick changes colour, then she will ovulate one to two days later. As some with PCOS have high levels of LH, then theoretically the LH-detection kit may sometimes be falsely positive. In practice, however, this rarely seems to be the case and most patients with PCOS find that these kits work well.

The progesterone blood test
Large amounts of the second female hormone, progesterone, are made after ovulation and this can be detected in a blood test. If you have a 28-day cycle, then a test is usually done on day 21. However, if you have a 35-day cycle, it has to be done later than day 21. Blood levels of progesterone peak seven days after ovulation, so the test is best linked with information from a BBTc and/or an ovulation detection kit. In the second half of the cycle, progesterone is released in large pulses, peaking every three hours. If the blood level of progesterone is higher than 20–30 nmol/L (6.3–9.4 ng/mL), ovulation is presumed to have occurred. Some centres use salivary levels of progesterone, rather than blood.

Lifestyle measures to improve fertility

As I shall discuss in the next chapter, a low-GI diet and plenty of exercise are likely to improve fertility. Time and time again, I have seen an overweight woman with PCOS conceive after she has lost just 4–5 kilograms (8–11 pounds). It is a good idea to commence this well before you plan to become pregnant, to reduce your risk of developing diabetes during pregnancy. The fitter you are, the lower your risk of developing this problem. Pregnancy diabetes, or gestational diabetes, is associated with an increased risk of foetal lung problems, intrauterine death and birth trauma, because the babies are often very large. Women with gestational diabetes also have a higher than usual risk of urinary infections, thrush and high blood pressure.

Medical treatments to improve fertility

If you are not ovulating, this is generally the easiest fertility problem to fix. Most overweight women with PCOS will start ovulating and then conceive with the lifestyle changes already discussed—weight loss, a low-GI diet and exercise are very likely to restore ovulation. However, some lose weight and still don't ovulate, and there are some thin women with an excellent lifestyle who have PCOS and don't ovulate, so they might need a drug therapy to help them. Some are keen to try a herbal therapy. Mills and Bone (2000) recommend herbals such as blue cohosh, agnus castus and helonias root to restore ovulation, but do not provide any scientific trials to support their recommendations.

Metformin to help with ovulation

Some women with insulin resistance respond to metformin therapy, which improves insulin resistance and aids weight loss. There is a lack of large-scale, properly conducted clinical trials on this drug, but the best information to date suggests that metformin (at a dose of 1.5–2 grams daily) restores ovulation in around 50 per cent of women with PCOS who are not ovulating. I am also concerned that there is a lack of information about foetal exposure. There is some information from South Africa, where metformin was used to treat a couple of hundred pregnant diabetic women, and those studies did not show an increased risk of foetal abnormalities. This is by no means conclusive, however. Generally, it is desirable to have safety information on a couple of thousand pregnancies before a drug is pronounced to be safe for use in pregnancy.

Dr Simmons and colleagues have reviewed the use of metformin during pregnancy (Simmons et al., 2004). They agreed that the currently available studies on metformin are not definitive but suggest that continuing metformin during pregnancy may reduce the risk of miscarriage, reduce the risk of gestational diabetes and seems to be associated with favourable pregnancy outcomes. They point out, however, that metformin does cross the placenta and therefore caution is advised. An Australian and New Zealand randomised controlled trial of metformin during pregnancy has commenced (the MiG trial). The trial aims to recruit 750 women over the next two years. The results of this trial are eagerly anticipated.

Some of my patients have used metformin in combination with a low-GI diet and exercise program, to lose weight and restore their cycle. I usually recommend they use condoms during this phase of their treatment and then, once they are ovulating regularly and the insulin resistance has improved, the metformin can be stopped and the lifestyle measures continued. Pregnancy usually occurs soon afterwards. If you are taking metformin, then the drug should be stopped as soon as the pregnancy is confirmed, unless you and your doctor have discussed the risks and have decided to continue the drug during pregnancy.

Clomiphene

The most commonly prescribed fertility drug is clomiphene. Clomiphene was discovered in 1956 when the search was on for a contraceptive Pill. It was first used clinically in the United States in 1967. It is an anti-oestrogen that tricks the brain into thinking that there isn't enough oestrogen around, so the pituitary releases more FSH, which in turn stimulates follicles to grow. It also sensitises the ovary to the effects of FSH. Basically, clomiphene amplifies the early hormonal events of the menstrual cycle. However, because clomiphene is an anti-oestrogen, it can have adverse fertility effects, particularly on the uterine lining and cervical mucus. It can bind to the oestrogen receptor for weeks. These adverse effects seem to be much more marked in women over the age of 35 years.

Around 80 per cent of women will ovulate with clomiphene, although only about half of them conceive. Most women around twenty years of age who are ovulating with clomiphene will conceive, whereas probably only around 10 per cent of those over the age of 35 years will get pregnant. In couples with no other fertility factors operating apart from failing to ovulate, the six-month pregnancy rate with clomiphene is between 30 and 50 per cent. Most conceptions occur in the first four cycles, and most researchers have found that, overall, about 30 to 50 per cent of women with PCOS will conceive on clomiphene within six cycles. If the therapy is continued for another six cycles, there will be only a few more pregnancies. Clomiphene-induced pregnancies do not have an increased risk of miscarriage, foetal abnormalities or antenatal problems.

Clomiphene should not be used as a long-term treatment to regulate cycles: a simple ovarian cyst can occur, plus clomiphene usually aggravates existing acne or excess hair. It is usually well tolerated, but side-effects include hot flushes (10 per cent), abdominal bloatedness (6 per cent), nausea (2 per cent) and headaches (1 per cent). The risk of twins is between 7 and 10 per cent; triplets or higher are rare.

For those who are clearly not ovulating, and since many pregnancies occur in the first three cycles, I usually delay other fertility tests until after three ovulatory cycles with clomiphene. The tests that I normally perform prior to starting clomiphene are:

- pre-pregnancy tests (e.g. check Rubella immunity);
- LH;
- FSH;
- TSH for thyroid function;
- prolactin;
- androgens;
- blood glucose and lipid levels.

Chapter 4 discussed the role of hormone measurements, but a couple of further points need to be made here. First, an abnormal blood result should always be repeated. Second, a raised FSH (more than 40 u/L or 40 mu/mL) suggests early menopause, which means fertility drugs simply won't work. Third, an abnormal TSH should prompt a full thyroid investigative screen. This usually involves a repeat TSH level as well as free T4, free T3, thyroid antibody levels and sometimes a thyroid scan. Fourth, a persistently elevated prolactin level should be investigated (see Chapter 4) and treated before using fertility drugs. Lastly, it is prudent to check blood lipids and glucose prior to starting fertility drugs in case there is any suggestion of insulin resistance. For those with insulin resistance, one of the major risks during pregnancy is developing diabetes.

It is prudent to check blood lipids and glucose prior to starting fertility drugs in case there is any suggestion of insulin resistance. For those with insulin resistance, one of the major risks during pregnancy is developing diabetes.

Patient story: Nathalie, 35 years old

Nathalie first came to see me because she needed help to get pregnant. She had been diagnosed with PCOS and had not had a period for three years (her pregnancy test was negative). Nathalie was overweight and we had a long chat about the importance of a low-GI, low-fat diet and exercise. She brought her blood hormone results with her, but she had not yet had her blood lipids or glucose checked. Her blood pressure was elevated at 160/95 mmHg (normal is around 120/80). There was a strong family history of late-onset diabetes, so I ordered a full glucose tolerance test as well as her lipids. Nathalie's test results are shown in Table 6.2.

Table 6.2 Nathalie's blood test results

	Fasting	One hour	Two hours
Blood glucose	5.2 mmol/L (3.4–5.4)	12	9.5 (<7.8)
	93.7 mg/dL (61.3–97.3)	216.2/171.2	(<140.5)
Blood insulin	18 mu/L (<12)	110 (<60)	323 (<60)
Cholesterol	7.5 mmol/L (<5.5)		
	289.6 mg/dL (<212.4)		
Triglycerides	5.0 mmol/L (<2)		
	442.5 mg/dL (<177)		

Note: Normal ranges are in brackets. Diabetic results would be a fasting glucose >6.9 mmol/L (>124.3 mg/dL) or a two-hour glucose >11 mmol/L (198.2 mg/dL).

The blood glucose levels are between the normal and diabetic ranges. Most experts describe this state as 'pre-diabetic', although the usual term used in this situation is 'impaired glucose tolerance'. High blood insulin levels, typical of insulin resistance, are seen here. Nathalie's cholesterol level of 7.5 mmol/L or 289.6 mg/dL (the normal level is <5.5 mmol/L or <212.4 mg/dL) and triglyceride level of 5.0 mmol/L or 442.5 mg/dL (<2.0 mmol/L or <177 mg/dL) are markedly elevated. She has Syndrome X, and if she conceived in this state she would almost certainly develop full-blown pregnancy-induced diabetes. I advised Nathalie to use contraception (condoms) until we had her metabolic state under control.

Using clomiphene

Some doctors like to intensively monitor every patient having ovulation induction, including clomiphene. This means having multiple blood tests and ultrasound scans—at considerable cost. As there are many pregnancies in the first three to four cycles of clomiphene, I prefer to start off simply—using temperature charts and a few blood tests. The usual starting dose of clomiphene is 50 milligrams for five days, starting on the second day of a natural or induced period. The following patient story illustrates the use of this drug.

Patient story: Karen, 28 years old

Karen had known PCOS and was referred to me for ovulation drugs. She only had one to two natural periods a year. Her BMI was normal and she was already on a low-GI, low-fat diet and had an excellent lifestyle. A pregnancy test was negative. I gave her ten days of a combined contraceptive Pill to induce a period. On day two of the induced period, she started clomiphene at 50 milligrams daily for five days. Karen also started taking her mouth temperature each morning and recording it on graph paper. I saw her five weeks later.

There was no clear rise in temperature, which would be expected after ovulation. Clearly the dose had not worked. I then prescribed a ten-day course of the Pill to bring on a period. This time she took 100 milligrams of clomiphene for five days. She had a period about a month later and she faxed me her temperature chart.

This time she had a sustained temperature rise in the second half of the cycle. I like to see at least a half-degree Celsius (one degree Fahrenheit) rise in temperature. I told her to take another course of 100 milligrams of clomiphene and this time we also tested her blood level of progesterone seven days after she ovulated, according to her chart. (Often there is a 'dip' on the chart at ovulation and then the temperature rises after that.) On that cycle, her blood progesterone was 85 nmol/L (26.7 ng/mL), which clearly confirmed she had ovulated (progesterone levels more than 20–30 nmol/L (6.3–9.4 ng/mL) are usually indicative of ovulation). This time her period was overdue, her temperature was still up four weeks after ovulation and a pregnancy test confirmed that Karen was indeed pregnant.

Patient story: Katie, 27 years old
Katie had conceived on clomiphene for her first pregnancy. She had PCOS and, despite being thin (her BMI was 20), Katie did not have spontaneous periods at all. Her blood test results are shown in Table 6.3.

Katie's tests are consistent with PCOS (high LH and testosterone) and there is no evidence of insulin resistance.

The raised blood levels of LH and testosterone and low SHBG levels are indicative of PCOS. I was reassured that her blood lipids and glucose were normal. I gave Katie a ten-day course of a contraceptive Pill to induce a period. On the second day, she started a five-day course of 50 milligrams of clomiphene. I initially monitored Katie's cycle with a temperature chart. Six weeks later, she had not had a period and was not pregnant. She took another ten-day course of the Pill to induce a period and this time she took 100 milligrams of clomiphene daily for five days. Again, she failed to ovulate. The third time around she took 150 milligrams of clomiphene for five days and I suggested that she use an LH-detection kit along with her temperature chart. Surprisingly, Katie did not ovulate with the 150 milligram dosage. I discussed some further options with her and she decided to try FSH therapy (see below). She conceived on her second FSH therapy cycle.

Table 6.3 Katie's blood test results

Hormone test	Katie's results	Normal range
LH, u/L	18	2–12
FSH	4.2	2–12
Prolactin, ng/mL	12	<20
TSH, mu/L	1.0	0.4–5.0
Testosterone, nmol/L (ng/dL)	3.5 (100.9)	1.5–2.6 (43.2–74.9)
SHBG, nmol/L (ng/dL)	22 (0.63)	20–120 (0.53–3.46)
DHEAS, umol/L (ng/mL)	7.9 (2910.8)	<11 (4053.1)
17-hydroxyprogesterone, nmol/L (g/L)	2 (0.7)	<6 (2)
Glucose, mmol/L (mg/dL)	4.5 (81.1)	3.4–5.4 (61.3–97.3)
Fasting insulin, mu/L	4	<12
Cholesterol, mmol/L (mg/dL)	3.6 (139)	<5.5 (212.4)
Triglycerides, mmol/L (mg/dL)	1.1 (97.3)	<2.0 (177)

Patient story: Sara, 25 years old
Sara had PCOS and she had lost 7 kilograms (15 pounds) in weight on a low-GI diet, but still wasn't ovulating. I suggested she take the contraceptive Pill for ten days and start on 50 milligrams of clomiphene daily for five days. Three weeks later, Sara came back to see me because of moderately severe pelvic pain. An ultrasound scan showed enlarged cystic ovaries consistent with mild hyperstimulation syndrome.

Often conception occurs in these cycles; however, this didn't occur in Sara's case and a week later she had her period. The cystic ovaries settled down after her period. Sara had a month off the clomiphene and again didn't ovulate. She then took the contraceptive Pill for ten days to bring on a period, and this time I suggested that she take 25 milligrams (half a 50 milligram tablet) of clomiphene daily for five days. Her temperature charts confirmed ovulation but she didn't conceive. I asked Sara to take the 25 milligram dose again for five days, starting from the second day of her period and she conceived.

A simple ovarian cyst occurs in around one in twenty cycles of clomiphene. This can often be ignored, but if it is very painful it is probably best to miss one cycle of clomiphene. Enlarged hyperstimulated ovaries are far less common, probably occurring in less than 1 per cent of clomiphene cycles. In these cases, it is best to avoid taking the drug until the pain has settled. Rarely, the pain can be so severe that the woman has to be admitted to hospital for pain relief and an intravenous drip.

What to do if clomiphene doesn't work
Those who fail to ovulate with clomiphene are usually offered metformin and clomiphene or FSH therapy next, although some may be offered ovarian diathermy. I will discuss both of these latter two treatments shortly. In the United States, very large doses of clomiphene—up to 250 milligrams for ten days—have been used and a few pregnancies have been reported. There have been reports of some success in combining clomiphene with dexamethasone (0.5 milligrams at night for ten days, starting on day two of the cycle). Dexamethasone suppresses the adrenal's production of androgens and in these doses side-effects are rare. Some specialists advocate the addition of a shot of human chorionic gonadotropin (hCG), a source of luteinising hormone (LH), five to seven days

after the clomiphene course. Clinical trials have mostly found that the addition of hCG didn't help the pregnancy rate.

Most women who fail to ovulate with clomiphene are best treated with FSH therapy, which is a highly successful treatment with few side-effects if it is closely monitored. There may be a role for stopping the clomiphene and focusing on further weight loss, metformin and exercise to improve the metabolic state, and then retrying the clomiphene.

Patient story: Tracey, 24 years old
Tracey had tried clomiphene, up to 150 milligrams for five days, and still wasn't ovulating. She was about 20 kilograms (44 pounds) overweight, but had already lost 15 kilograms (33 pounds). Rather than giving her stronger medication, I suggested she have some time out from drug treatment to focus further on lifestyle factors. She added a couple of gym workouts to her exercise regimen, continued on her low-GI diet and over the next six months lost another 6 kilograms (13 pounds), but still didn't conceive. I asked her to retry the clomiphene and this time she conceived using only the 50 milligram dose for five days.

FSH therapy
FSH therapy is a highly successful therapy for women who are not ovulating due to PCOS. There are several preparations available, as summarised in Table 6.4.

For over 30 years, a product derived from the urine of menopausal women (human menopausal gonadotrophin, or hMG) has been the major FSH therapy. Each ampoule of hMG contains 75 units of FSH and 75 units of LH, as well as some proteins (which can cause the occasional allergic reaction). These products are not orally active and have to be given by injection into the muscle. The newer products are pure FSH without the protein contamination, so they can be given as a subcutaneous injection—that is, just under the skin rather than deep into the muscle. A small 'pen' injector, similar to the one people with diabetes have used for years, is now available for FSH injections. These devices allow the woman to give her own injection, using a smaller volume of fluid than with conventional FSH therapy.

Table 6.4 Types of FSH therapy

Preparation	Trade names
Human menopausal	Humegon, Menogon,
gonadotrophins	Pergonal, Repronex
Purified urinary FSH	Normegon, Metrodyn, Orgafol
Highly purified urinary FSH	Metrodin HP, Fertinex
Recombinant FSH	Gonal-F, Follistim, Puregon
Human chorionic	Pregnyl, Profasi, APL
gonadotrophin	
Recombinant hCG (rhCG)	Ovidrel
Recombinant LH (rLH)	Lhadi

It is important that other fertility factors are checked prior to initiating FSH treatment. Apart from measuring hormone levels (if the FSH level is more than 20 u/L (20 mu/mL), this indicates menopause or a perimenopausal state, and FSH therapy is useless in these cases), the fallopian tubes are assessed by performing a laparoscopy or a hysterosalpingoram (HSG), which involves passing a dye through the cervix into the tubes to check that there are no blockages. The woman's partner should also have his sperm count and motility checked as well.

Using FSH therapy
There are many ways of using FSH therapy, but the method outlined below is one of the main ones used. Treatment is usually started after a natural or induced period; otherwise an ultrasound scan is performed to demonstrate that the uterine lining is thin and

there are no large ovarian cysts prior to commencing ovulation induction. Periodic ultrasound scans and/or blood oestradiol levels are performed to monitor the follicular response. FSH therapy usually begins by giving one ampoule of FSH daily for seven days. Those with PCOS tend to be sensitive to FSH treatment, so some experts start with just half an ampoule of FSH and give that for fourteen days before increasing the dose. Further increases occur at seven-day intervals.

Once there is clear follicular growth on ultrasound with rising levels of blood oestradiol, the dose of FSH is kept constant. Generally, once there is a dominant follicle of 10 millimetres (0.39 inches) in diameter, it will double its size in five days without increasing the FSH dosage. If FSH dosage is increased at this point, more follicles will grow. Once the lead follicle(s) have reached a diameter of 18–20 millimetres (0.71–0.78 inches) and blood oestradiol levels are around 1000 pmol/L (272.4 pg/mL) per follicle, the FSH treatment is stopped and a single injection of 250 micrograms of rhCG is given to trigger ovulation—which is similar to what the LH surge would naturally do. If there are more than four follicles larger than 14 millimetres (0.55 inches), or if the blood oestradiol level is greater than 8000 to 10 000 pmol/L (2179.2–2724 pg/mL), then generally the rhCG is withheld as there is a significant risk of hyperstimulation of the ovaries. If the rhCG is given, then ovulation usually occurs about 36 hours later. The couple is encouraged to have sex 24 to 36 hours after the rhCG shot.

If a cycle of therapy has produced numerous large follicles, then another approach is adopted by some units. This involves giving the rhCG injection and performing IVF. The woman is given a light anaesthetic and the eggs are collected using an ultrasound-guided needle. The eggs are fertilised using the partner's sperm and the resulting embryos are frozen. In this case, the couple abstains from sex so that natural conception doesn't occur, hopefully avoiding hyperstimulation. The embryos are then transferred during another cycle using natural hormones to prepare the uterus, rather than FSH. Often eight to twenty eggs can be obtained on these cycles. Unfortunately egg quality can be poor if more than 15 eggs are collected and so a smaller number of embryos may be available to freeze and store. Depending on the age of the woman, one to three embryos will be placed back into the uterus, resulting in a pregnancy rate of around 20–30 per cent per embryo transfer.

Results of FSH therapy

If a woman's only fertility problem is lack of ovulation, then FSH therapy is highly successful, having a cumulative pregnancy rate of 50–60 per cent after six cycles of treatment. Dr Graeme Hughes has been running the FSH program at the Royal Hospital for Women in Sydney for many years. In over 90 per cent of cycles, ovulation has occurred and the monthly conception rate was 20–25 per cent, which is comparable to the normal background pregnancy rate in the general population. There have been numerous medical papers published on FSH treatment (e.g. Ludwig et al., 2003; Dale et al., 1992). According to the world literature on FSH therapy, the chance of multiple births is between 10 and 30 per cent, with most of these being twins. The normal risk of twins is one in 80, or around 1 per cent. There is no increased risk of miscarriage with FSH therapy—unless a multiple pregnancy occurs. Keep in mind that as a woman approaches 40 years of age the miscarriage rate starts to approach 40 per cent, even in the normal population.

FSH therapy is associated with a 1–2 per cent risk of ovarian hyperstimulation, which is a very serious complication of ovulation induction therapy. In mild cases, the swollen ovaries produce mild abdominal swelling and pain with some degree of fluid retention. The condition usually resolves with simple analgesics such as paracetamol and plenty of fluids. The hyperstimulated ovaries are fragile and can bleed easily, so rest is advised and sexual intercourse should be avoided until the condition settles as the enlarged ovaries can be bumped during sex. In severe cases, however, the ovaries become greatly enlarged with large multiple follicles and swelling. There is usually severe abdominal pain and distention. Fluid moves from the circulation into the abdominal cavity, so the blood becomes concentrated and thick, which can cause blood clots and shock. Such affected women need to be admitted to hospital and given intravenous fluids and closely monitored. It is important to keep in mind that the condition is self-limiting: if conception doesn't occur, the syndrome usually resolves itself within seven days; on the other hand, if pregnancy occurs then hyperstimulation may continue for two to four weeks.

Patient story: Amanda, 34 years old

Amanda had PCOS and failed to ovulate with clomiphene, so she decided to try FSH therapy. A baseline ultrasound scan showed a normal-sized uterus and a thin uterine lining. She started taking one ampoule of FSH daily. A week later, a scan showed no follicular growth, so the dosage of FSH was increased to two ampoules daily. Five days later, a scan showed two follicles, each around 10 millimetres (0.39 inches) in size, and her blood oestradiol level was 472 pmol/L (128.6 pg/mL). The dosage was kept at two ampoules daily. Another five days later, the two follicles were now 18–22 millimetres (0.71–0.87 inches) in size and her blood oestradiol was 2271 pmol/L (618.6 pg/mL), so the FSH was stopped and rhCG were given. Amanda made sure that she and her partner had sex 24 and 36 hours later. She conceived on that cycle and had a normal, uneventful pregnancy.

Patient story: Danielle, 28 years old

Danielle was a thin woman with PCOS. She had just one period per year on average. Her blood test results are shown in Table 6.5.

Danielle had a good diet and exercise program, but still wasn't ovulating. She tried clomiphene up to 150 milligrams for five days without success, then moved on to FSH therapy. A baseline scan showed a normal-sized uterus but a rather thick uterine lining, so she was given the contraceptive Pill to take for three weeks. She then had a period and started on FSH therapy, at one ampoule daily. A week later, another scan showed no follicular growth and her blood oestradiol level was low. The dosage was therefore increased to two ampoules daily. A week later, the scan showed four follicles around 10 millimetres (0.39 inches) in size and a blood oestradiol level of 950 pmol/L (258.8 pg/mL). Her dosage was kept at two ampoules daily. Four days later, a scan showed six follicles between 14 and 16 millimetres (0.55–0.63 inches) in diameter and a blood oestradiol level of 5243 pmol/L (1428.2 pg/mL), so the cycle was abandoned for fear of producing either ovarian hyperstimulation or a multiple birth.

Danielle again took the Pill for three weeks and then recommenced FSH therapy. This time she was given one ampoule for fourteen days. At the end of that time she had two follicles, each 10 millimetres (0.39 inches) in diameter, and her blood oestradiol level was 600 pmol/L (163.4 pg/mL). The dosage was kept at one ampoule daily. Three days later, the follicles had grown in size to 15–16 millimetres (0.59–0.63 inches) and her blood oestradiol level was 1245 pmol/L (339.1 pg/mL). A few days later, both follicles were larger than 18 millimetres (0.71 inches) in size and her blood oestradiol level was just over 2000 pmol/L (544.8 pg/mL), so the FSH was stopped and rhCG was given. She did not conceive during that cycle, but she did fall pregnant on the third cycle of FSH therapy, following a similar regimen.

Table 6.5 Danielle's blood test results

Hormone result	Danielle's results	Normal range
LH, u/L	10	2–12
FSH, u/L (mu/mL)	4.4 (4.4)	2–12 (2–12)
Prolactin, ng/mL	7	<20
TSH, mu/L	1.7	0.4–5.0
Testosterone, nmol/L (ng/dL)	3.8 (109.5)	1.5–2.6 (43.2–74.9)
SHBG, nmol/L (ng/dL)	29 (0.84)	20–120 (0.58–3.46)
DHEAS, umol/L (ng/mL)	9.1 (3353)	<11 (4053.1)
17-hydroxyprogesterone, nmol/L (g/L)	4 (1.3)	<6 (2)
Glucose, mmol/L (mg/dL)	4.2 (75.7)	3.4–5.4 (61.3–97.3)
Fasting insulin, mu/L	10	<12
Cholesterol, mmol/L (mg/dL)	3.1 (119.7)	<5.5 (<212.4)
Triglycerides, mmol/L (mg/dL)	0.7 (61.9)	<2.0 (<177)

Surgical treatments to improve fertility

In the past, an operation called a 'wedge-resection' was performed in an attempt to reduce the size of the ovaries. This involved removing a piece of each ovary—much like taking a slice out of a small melon—and then stitching up the defect in the ovary. Dr Stein, a US gynaecologist who pioneered the operation, found that amongst the 108 cases that he operated on, 95 per cent of the women started to have regular menstrual cycles again and 87 per cent conceived (see Stein, 1956). The initial interest in the surgical approach waned when it was found that the operation often produced significant adhesions, and further decreased once drug therapies became available, as they were preferred over surgery. In the past decade or so, there has been renewed interest in the surgical approach, with the advent of laparoscopic surgery—particularly with PCOS women.

Laparoscopic surgery for PCOS
Laparoscopy involves a small telescope being passed through a small incision near the navel, under general anaesthetic. This permits the surgeon to inspect the pelvic contents such as the uterus, fallopian tubes and ovaries. The most common laparoscopic operation for PCOS is called an 'ovarian diathermy'. This usually involves making a series of burns (four to eight) in each of the ovaries with either an electrical current or using laser. In 1989, Dr Gjonnaess reported on a group of 190 women with PCOS who underwent laparoscopic ovarian diathermy. He found that 89 of the women conceived with only a 15 per cent miscarriage rate. There have been many published reports since then with similar results (e.g. Farquhar et al., 2002). However, the risk of complications seems a little unclear (Greenblatt and Casper, 1993).

Theoretically, damage to the ovaries can result in scarring and adhesions around the ovaries and tubes, and may also bring on early menopause because of a loss of follicles. Some reports show a high rate of pelvic adhesions (e.g. Greenblatt and Casper, 1993). However, the quality of the follow-up after surgery varies tremendously from study to study. The adhesions can only be diagnosed by performing a second laparoscopy some months later, and most of the published studies have not done this. I am not aware of any long-term studies examining the risk of early menopause. In my opinion, the lack of decent follow-up information makes laparoscopic surgery a second-line option to drugs for ovulation induction.

All this does beg the question: why does injury to the ovary stimulate ovulation? The size of the injury seems to correlate with the duration of the effect. In the mid-1980s, I was involved in some research studying the hormonal content of ovarian follicular fluid in both normal and polycystic ovaries (Eden 1989). This research involved placing a needle into the follicles to collect the fluid. Simply aspirating follicles from the ovary seems to induce a few ovulations, although usually only one to three. The effect of laparoscopic diathermy seems to last around one to three years, whereas a wedge resection seems to produce regular cycles for some years. Research has shown that laparoscopic surgery results in lower blood androgen and LH levels, but often these changes are short-lived. The ovarian injury seems to sensitise the ovaries to FSH, and it has been postulated that the injury alters the intra-ovarian controls in some way, making the ovaries respond better to FSH.

Patient story: Ghada, 25 years old
Ghada had PCOS and developed marked ovarian hyperstimulation on a very low dose of FSH treatment. She required hospitalisation and was understandably scared to have further ovulation induction. She underwent laparoscopic ovarian diathermy. All went well and her cycles normalised. Ghada conceived on her fourth natural cycle.

In summary, laparoscopic surgery has some advantages and disadvantages over drug therapies for inducing ovulation. These are summarised in Table 6.6.

Table 6.6 Laparoscopic surgery to induce ovulation

Laparoscopic surgery	Fertility drugs
High pregnancy rate	High pregnancy rate
Lower risk of miscarriage than fertility drugs	
Risks of surgery and anaesthetic	No anaesthetic needed
No risk of hyperstimulation	A 1–2 per cent risk of hyper-stimulation
No monitoring needed	Intensive monitoring required
Risk of adhesions and early menopause	No surgical risks
Single treatment	Multiple treatments needed

Do PCO and PCOS affect pregnancy outcomes?

Once a woman is pregnant, she may fear the worst. Most women will carry their babies through to birth without complication; however, there are some statistics that do show a slightly higher risk of miscarriage and gestational diabetes for women with PCOS. We will now examine the risks in more detail and discuss ways to minimise these complications (Norman et al., 2004; Eden and Warren, 1999).

Miscarriage

Overall, around 15 per cent of clinical pregnancies result in miscarriage. (Clinical pregnancy means that you are sufficiently far along to know that you are pregnant.) Around 1 per cent of women have recurrent miscarriages, meaning three or more. These women seem to have a high rate of scan evidence of PCO, although many of them will have fairly regular menstrual cycles and don't fit the definition of PCOS. Several studies have shown a link between blood levels of LH and risk of miscarriage. Around half of all women with PCOS will have raised blood levels of LH, at least on one occasion.

There have been several explanations for why high LH levels may cause miscarriages. One animal study has shown that high LH levels can cause premature egg ageing, resulting in reduced fertilisation and increased risk of a poor-quality embryo (see reference in Eden, 1989). High LH also stimulates ovarian androgen production, which may in turn affect ovarian function or even the lining of the uterus. GnRH drugs suppress the pituitary release of LH and FSH and can be given in conjunction with FSH therapy to produce a low-LH environment. Clinical trials using these approaches have produced conflicting results. One placebo-controlled trial by Dr Clifford and colleagues (1996) showed that GnRH treatment was no better than placebo at preventing miscarriages, even though the GnRH treatment successfully suppressed blood LH levels. In summary, the idea that high LH levels cause miscarriage sounds interesting, but at the moment lacks hard evidence.

One Australian study by Dr Anne Clark (Clark et al., 1998) showed that weight loss not only increases the rate of ovulation amongst women with PCOS, but also reduces the risk of miscarriage. As already discussed, laparoscopic ovarian diathermy often restores ovulations in women with PCOS and is associated with a miscarriage rate that is similar to that of the background population (around 15 per cent).

Pregnancy-induced diabetes

Pregnancy often induces a temporary diabetic state—so-called gestational diabetes, which usually affects 5–10 per cent of all pregnancies. The risk varies tremendously according to the population studied. Some racial groups, such as Asians, seem to have a higher risk due to genetic factors, although a high-GI diet is likely to contribute to this. There are few studies available at the moment that examine the risk of gestational diabetes amongst women with

PCOS, but those that have been published suggest a slightly higher risk of diabetes during pregnancy for those with PCOS (Norman et al., 2004). Normally, being overweight is a risk factor for diabetes, but that doesn't seem to apply to women with PCOS. Both overweight and thin women with PCOS can have insulin resistance, and this can be expected to worsen during pregnancy.

Fortunately, most cases of gestational diabetes are mild and have little effect on mother and child. However, severe gestational diabetes can be associated with a number of pregnancy complications, including obstructed labour due to a large baby and lung problems for the baby. Those women who have gestational diabetes are at increased risk of developing full-blown diabetes later in life. As I will discuss in the next chapter, a low-GI diet and exercise have been shown to reduce the risk of diabetes by around 60 per cent.

Summary

Fertility issues are a major concern for women with PCOS. Many women with PCOS will conceive naturally. A low-GI, low-fat diet combined with a vigorous exercise program promotes both ovulation and conception, and tends to prevent miscarriage. Many women ovulate infrequently, rather than not at all. Those women who are sexually active but don't wish to conceive still need to use contraception—for most women with PCOS a combined contraceptive Pill will be the best option as it helps with menstrual control and usually helps considerably with the skin problems such as excess hair and acne. However, it might be necessary to watch blood lipid levels. Sometimes the triglyceride levels, in particular, can rise due to the oestrogen component of the Pill. The Mirena device will be a good option for others. It combines excellent contraception with menstrual control and has little or no impact on blood factors such as triglyceride levels. The Mirena device also lowers the risk of pelvic infection, lasts for five years and has the benefit that fertility returns immediately upon removing the device.

When women with PCOS want to have a baby, some may fail to ovulate regularly. They are usually offered the drug clomiphene to induce ovulation. Around 80 per cent of women will ovulate with clomiphene, although only about half will conceive. This is because clomiphene is an anti-oestrogen and so can have adverse fertility effects on the cervical mucus and uterine lining. These adverse effects are more marked in older women. However, despite this, clomiphene is a simple, very useful and successful treatment for women with PCOS.

For those who fail to respond to clomiphene, there are three main options: metformin and clomiphene, FSH therapy or surgery. FSH, a pituitary hormone that stimulates follicles to grow, is a highly effective treatment—the monthly conception rate is similar to that of a normal population. FSH therapy does need to be closely monitored to avoid multiple ovulations, which may result in multiple births and occasionally ovarian hyperstimulation syndrome. Ovarian wedge resection was the original surgery option offered to women with PCOS, and was successful at achieving pregnancies. It also had significant risks, however, including adhesions and a large abdominal incision, so it fell out of favour. In the past decade or so, laparoscopic operations on the polycystic ovaries have received some attention because ovulation can often be restored with a low miscarriage rate. However, there is little information on long-term complications, such as adhesions and early menopause.

Frequently asked questions

I was told that I am infertile because I have PCOS. Is that true?

No. Dr Dahlgren's Swedish research (Dahlgren et al., 1992) showed that 76 per cent of women with PCOS in her study had at least one baby. This agrees with my experience, which is that many women with PCOS will conceive naturally. Weight loss, a low-GI diet and exercise all help. For those who continue not to ovulate, despite a good diet and exercise, fertility drugs are very successful.

I am 28 years old, have PCOS and am sexually active. Do I need contraception?

Yes!

I'm scared to take the Pill because it might stop me having children later. Is that true?

No. The Pill actually preserves fertility by lowering the risk of some diseases that can cause fertility problems. The risk of pelvic infections, endometriosis, ovarian cysts and fibroids are all lower for Pill users. Only around 1 per cent of women will not menstruate once they come off the Pill, which is comparable to the general population. In my experience, these women usually have PCOS and have gained weight over the preceding years. A low-fat, low-GI diet usually restores the cycle.

I'm 39 years old and normally have two periods a year with PCOS. I'm currently on a contraceptive Pill but I smoke 20 cigarettes a day. Which is the best contraceptive for me?

Stop smoking! If you don't stop smoking then you should stop the Pill because of the increased health risks involved. Try a different contraceptive method. Alternatives include condoms, a diaphragm, Implanon or a Mirena device

I don't ovulate because of PCOS but I'm trying to have a baby. Clomiphene didn't work for me and I tried FSH therapy but developed severe hyperstimulation syndrome. Now I'm scared to take FSH again. What are my options?

There are a few other options. You could re-try clomiphene, this time adding dexamethasone. Another option could be to try metformin alone first, then perhaps with clomiphene. Lastly, diathermy of the ovaries using laparoscopic surgery is also worth considering.

7
Taking the sugar:
The diet and insulin story

While we do not know what causes PCOS, one of the great discoveries of the last few years has been the uncovering of the link between sugar, insulin and PCOS. Biologically, it makes complete sense that nutritional factors should impact on fertility. If a woman doesn't have her dietary factors right, then it is not a good time for her to get pregnant, as the foetus may be adversely affected. Weight is another factor that can influence reproduction. If you are too thin, your periods will stop; conversely, if you gain too much weight then your periods can also stop. As we have already discussed, those with PCOS tend to stop ovulating if they gain weight. In contrast, those with 'normal ovaries' usually lose ovulations if they lose weight. Inadequate dietary protein intake will also slow the cycle. Thus it is no great surprise that energy intake (sugar and carbohydrates) might impact on the menstrual cycle too. Understanding how lifestyle factors such as diet and exercise can impact on PCOS is a major key to controlling symptoms.

Understanding how lifestyle factors such as diet and exercise can impact on PCOS is a major key to controlling symptoms.

What is insulin resistance?

Insulin is made by the pancreas, a gland that sits near the stomach (see Figure 1.2). It secretes both insulin and glucagon, two protein hormones, into the bloodstream from clumps of cells called 'the islets of Langerhans'. The pancreas also releases enzymes into the small bowel to aid digestion—especially the absorption of dietary sugars. Our discussion here will focus on the actions of insulin.

Insulin is normally released in response to rising blood glucose levels. The main function of insulin is to stimulate the uptake of glucose by cells, reducing the amount of glucose in the blood. Glucagon has almost the reverse effect. The secretion of both of these hormones is controlled by the amount of glucose in the blood. Insulin also has an important effect on blood fat levels, especially triglycerides. Some individuals appear to be insulin resistant (IR), which means that their tissues require higher than usual levels of insulin to function normally. Not all tissues are IR: the problem seems to reside mostly in the muscle and liver. Some parts of the body, such as the ovaries, are normally sensitive to insulin. We do not know why different parts of the body vary in their sensitivity to insulin.

Studies of individuals with IR (e.g. Dunaif, 1997) have shown that the insulin in their bloodstream and their insulin receptors seem to function normally, but that they have a problem handling insulin after it has attached to its receptor. The late-onset type 2 adult diabetes is associated with severe IR and often runs in families. Thus genetics can play a role, but often it is weight gain and the wrong type of diet that aggravate IR. Such affected individuals paradoxically have high blood insulin levels (to help their liver and muscles to process glucose), but still don't have enough insulin to lower their blood glucose levels.

It turns out that insulin also acts on the ovary to make more testosterone. Women must make testosterone first and then convert some of this androgen into the main female hormone, oestrogen. However, many women with PCOS have high blood insulin levels, which in turn act on their polycystic ovaries to over-produce testosterone. High insulin levels also seem to lower SHBG levels, leading to even higher free, bioactive testosterone levels. Rising testosterone levels act as a brake on the menstrual cycle and, in vulnerable individuals, can lead to excess body hair and acne. Insulin is a fat-promoting hormone. As such, those with IR tend to gain weight, which in turn increases IR, producing a vicious cycle (see Figure 7.1). Therefore diet can play an important role in both the causes and the effects of PCOS.

Diagnosing IR

There is still considerable controversy about the best way to diagnose IR. I have no doubt that the scientist who solves the problem of IR should receive the Nobel Prize, but at the moment the precise cause of IR remains elusive. I suspect, however, that there are a number of ways to induce IR.

It is now well accepted that IR is a major cause of the so-called 'metabolic syndrome' or Syndrome X. The main features of this are obesity around the abdomen, raised blood triglycerides and cholesterol levels, and IR. Both men and women with Syndrome X are at increased risk of hypertension, diabetes and heart disease.

There are other visible signs of IR, such as the small number of people (1–5 per cent) with IR who have a particular skin condition called 'acanthosis nigricans'—a dark, velvety skin condition most commonly found on the back of the neck, in the

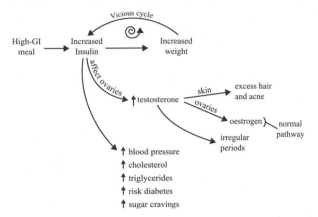

Figure 7.1 The impact of IR and excessively raised insulin levels

armpits and under the breasts. This is a direct result of the high insulin levels, and usually fades with successful treatment. Some of my patients with acanthosis thought that they had dirty skin in their armpits and were dismayed that they couldn't scrub it off! Only a minority of people with IR have acanthosis, however, so its absence does not mean that IR is not present. Some other signs of IR include:

- *metabolic indicators*:
  - high triglyceride levels;
  - high blood pressure;
  - increased risk of cardiovascular disease;
- *hormonal indicators*: high blood insulin levels leading to:
  - increased ovarian production of androgens;
  - lowered liver production of SHBG;
  - increased serum androgens;
  - altered secretion of LH;
  - infrequent ovulations;
- skin conditions such as:
  - acanthosis nigricans.

The Rotterdam Consensus PCOS Workshop Group (2004) defined the metabolic syndrome as being present in those with PCOS if three out of the following five indicators were present:

- waist circumference more than 88 centimetres (35 inches);
- raised blood triglyceride levels;
- low blood levels of HDL-cholesterol;
- raised blood pressure (top reading more than 130 mmHg or lower reading more than 85 mmHg);
- raised fasting or two-hour blood glucose levels from a 75 gram oral glucose tolerance test.

Blood tests

When diagnosing IR through blood tests, some doctors rely on fasting blood levels of glucose and insulin, and some on a glucose tolerance test (measuring both glucose and insulin levels over two hours). Others calculate ratios of insulin and glucose (called a homeostasis model assessment (HOMA)). If a fasting insulin level is used to diagnose IR, then three blood samples should be taken over ten minutes and averaged. Fasting insulin levels between 10 and 14 milliunits per litre (mu/L) probably indicate mild IR, whereas levels above 14 mu/L suggest more severe IR. A HOMA is calculated as follows:

$$\frac{\text{average of three fasting insulin levels (mu/L)} \times \text{fasting glucose (mmol/L)}}{22.5}$$

HOMA values less than 2.0 are normal, values between 2.0 and 3.0 suggest mild IR and above 3.0 probably indicates moderate to severe IR.

If I suspect a patient has IR, I usually order a glucose tolerance test (GTT), which measures both blood glucose and insulin levels. This test involves consuming a high-carbohydrate diet for a couple of days leading up to the test. On the day of the test, a fasting blood sample is collected, then the subject is given 75 grams of glucose in water to drink. Blood samples are taken one and two hours later. This tests the body's reaction to a glucose load. Normal blood glucose and insulin levels tend to peak and trough together. Those with IR tend to have inappropriately elevated and sustained levels of insulin (see Figure 7.2). One of the main reasons I like the GTT is that it reflects reality and allows me to find out how that particular woman's body reacts to a sugar load. A peak insulin level greater than 60 mu/L at one or two hours is probably indicative of insulin resistance. Some examples of this test follow in Tables 7.1–7.5.

Table 7.1 Glucose tolerance test 1 results

Subject 1	Fasting level	One hour after glucose drink	Two hours after glucose drink
Blood glucose, mmol/L (mg/dL)	4.0 (72.1)	6.0 (108.1)	4.2 (75.7)
Blood insulin, mu/L	4	30	7

Subject 1 shows a normal result on the glucose tolerance test. Blood glucose levels should be less than 5.5 mmol/L (99.1 mg/dL) after fasting and be less than 7.8 mmol/L (140.5 mg/dL) two hours after drinking glucose water. Blood insulin levels should be less than 12 mu/L at fasting, rising by four- to tenfold at one hour after drinking the glucose water, then falling to fasting levels two to four hours after the oral glucose load.

Table 7.2 Glucose tolerance test 2 results

Subject 2	Fasting level	One hour after glucose drink	Two hours after glucose drink
Blood glucose, mmol/L (mg/dL)	4.0 (72.1)	8.4 (151.3)	6.7 (120.7)
Blood insulin, mu/L	23	154	250

Subject 2 has a non-diabetic result, but the levels are consistent with insulin resistance. The blood glucose response to the oral glucose load is normal. However, fasting blood insulin levels are high, and continue to rise even two hours after the oral glucose load. This 'extra insulin' may cause sugar cravings and will promote the movement of sugar into fat cells, thereby increasing weight.

Table 7.3 Glucose tolerance test 3 results

Subject 3	Fasting level	One hour after glucose drink	Two hours after glucose drink
Blood glucose, mmol/L (mg/dL)	8 (144.1)	14 (252.3)	13 (234.2)
Blood insulin, mu/L	56	257	320

Subject 3 shows a diabetic result. The fasting blood glucose level is elevated (more than 6.9 mmol/L or 124.3 mg/dL), as is the two-hour blood glucose (more than 11 mmol/L or 198.2 mg/dL). High blood insulin levels are typical of overt type 2 diabetes.

Table 7.4 Glucose tolerance test 4 results

Subject 4	Fasting level	One hour after glucose drink	Two hours after glucose drink
Blood glucose, mmol/L (mg/dL)	5.7 (102.7)	11 (198.2)	10.0 (180.2)
Blood insulin, mu/L	35	120	270

Subject 4 has impaired glucose tolerance. These blood glucose levels are between normal and diabetic. Some authorities describe this state as 'pre-diabetic', although the usual term in this situation is 'impaired glucose tolerance'. High blood insulin levels, typical of insulin resistance, are seen.

The GTT accurately assesses blood glucose response to an oral glucose load. The insulin response is less accurate. The HOMA test is also fallible. As such it is important that these tests are interpreted as part of the overall assessment.

Table 7.5 Glucose tolerance test 5 results

Subject 5	Fasting level	One hour after glucose drink	Two hours after glucose drink	Three hours after glucose drink	Four hours after glucose drink
Blood glucose, mmol/L (mg/dL)	4.8 (86.5)	10 (180.2)	6.1 (109.9)	2.7 (48.6)	4.5 (81.1)
Blood insulin, mu/L	27	273	356	132	21

Some women with PCOS have sugar cravings after a meal and become very shaky, cold and sweaty around two to four hours after they have eaten. These symptoms suggest that they may be experiencing low blood glucose levels. In these cases, I usually ask them to have an extended GTT—four hours rather than two hours—to see if they are experiencing delayed hypoglycaemia (low blood sugar levels). Subject 5's results illustrate this point. Normally blood glucose and insulin levels rise and fall in a similar pattern. However, Subject 5 has clear evidence of IR—even her fasting blood insulin levels are raised, but she is not diabetic (her fasting and two hour blood glucose levels are normal). Two hours after the glucose drink, her blood glucose is back to normal, but she still has a markedly raised blood insulin level (356 mu/l) and this drives her blood glucose down to a very low level at three hours (2.7 mmol/l or 48.6 mg/dL). This could make her feel terrible—shaky, fatigued and dizzy. Things are getting back towards normal at four hours.

In summary, to detect IR, the minimum tests required are fasting blood glucose, insulin and blood fats (cholesterol and triglycerides). If bouts of low blood glucose or diabetes are suspected, the best test is a GTT, taking samples hourly for two to four hours after drinking 75 grams of glucose in water.

How do I control and prevent insulin resistance?

Even small amounts of weight loss (4–5 kilograms or 8–11 pounds) and/or modest amounts of exercise (three to four hours per week) can reverse IR, leading to an improved metabolic and hormonal profile, and usually more frequent ovulations. Controlling cholesterol and triglyceride levels and eating more omega-3 fatty acids (e.g. fish oils) have been shown to help. As a last resort, there are drugs available to help lower IR.

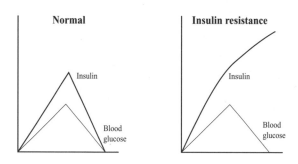

Figure 7.2 Insulin resistance

The weight of it

Twenty years ago, I noticed that many of my very overweight patients with PCOS started to ovulate more or less immediately on commencing a weight-loss diet. The interesting thing was that their cycles seemed to return before they had actually lost any significant amount of weight. In the past few years, the reason for this phenomenon has become apparent—it depended on the glycaemic index (GI) of the food they were eating.

Most weight-loss diets focus on low-fat foods, typically recommending less than 30 grams (1 ounce) of fat daily. The main reason for this approach is that fat contains twice as much energy as carbohydrates or protein on a weight-by-weight basis. However, many of my patients gained weight on low-fat diets. The problem with focusing on just a low-fat diet is that it will probably end up being too high in carbohydrates.

Carbohydrates are sugars, and they are an essential fuel for our body. There are many types, ranging from simple one-sugar molecules (monosaccharides) to complex sugar chains (polysaccharides). Before GI came along, it was thought that simple sugars were absorbed very quickly whereas polysaccharides were absorbed much more slowly. It turns out that it is the rate of emptying of the stomach that is the single most important factor that determines the rate of sugar absorption.

How the body digests and absorbs carbohydrates
Digestion starts in the mouth, where food is chewed into smaller pieces and mixed with amylase, an enzyme that breaks long sugar chains into shorter ones. However, once the food is swallowed and passes into the stomach, acids neutralise the amylase. No sugar is absorbed in the stomach. How fast the food passes out of the stomach is determined by some of the other components of the food. Fibre, acidity and highly concentrated solutions slow the emptying of the stomach, so they slow the speed of carbohydrate digestion. Most sugars are absorbed in the small bowel where large amounts of amylase are released. Here, most carbohydrates are rapidly absorbed; however some are relatively resistant to amylase and so they take longer to be digested.

Our body burns food components in a particular order. Alcohol goes first because it cannot be stored in the body, then protein, then carbohydrate and last is fat. Thus, if a large amount of alcohol is consumed with a meal, the body will probably burn the alcohol and store the meal as fat. Also, our body can burn only a limited amount of protein, so a high-protein diet will often result in weight loss, but this can be quite stressful on the body. The high-protein approach is the basis of the Scarsdale and Atkins diets. Basically, only sugar—which is converted into fat and dietary fats—can be stored in our fat cells.

Myth: All foods are processed the same way in the body. **Fact:** Our bodies burn food components differently and in the following order: alcohol, protein, carbohydrate and fat.

How insulin controls fat and sugars in our body
In the average diet, carbohydrates and fat are burnt by our bodies mostly for fuel. Our bodies then store any unused fat (i.e. fat we haven't burnt), resulting in weight gain. The hormone insulin, as well as aiding the absorption of sugar into our bodies, largely determines the amount of dietary fat or carbohydrate that is burnt by our bodies. Rapidly rising blood glucose levels result in high insulin levels. Conversely, slowly rising blood glucose levels induce slowly rising insulin levels. If insulin levels are low, then dietary fat is burnt in preference to sugar. On the other hand, if insulin levels are high, then carbohydrate is preferentially burnt.

People with IR have chronically high levels of insulin so their cells are constantly burning sugar in preference to fat. The unused dietary fat is then stored and weight gain results. The precise cause of insulin resistance remains a mystery, but in most cases genetics plays a role and lack of exercise, being overweight and a high-GI diet all contribute. Whatever the cause, insulin resistance results in chronically high blood insulin levels. This in turn will encourage the storage of fat and reduce fat burning, and is associated with high blood triglyceride levels (a type of fat found in the bloodstream) and high blood pressure.

All these factors will increase the risk of heart and blood vessel disease, stroke and diabetes. Exercise and a low-GI diet significantly lower the risk of diabetes. One large study examined a group of people who were at high risk of developing diabetes because of a strong family history of the disease. Three hours or more a week of exercise and a low-GI diet reduced the risk of diabetes by 60 per cent.

How GI levels are calculated

The glycaemic index, or GI, was first proposed by professors Jenkins and Wolever from the University of Toronto in 1981 (Jenkins et al., 1981). GI describes how much a particular food raises blood glucose levels. In other words, it is like a glucose tolerance test (GTT), but the effect of a portion of food rather than a pure sugar drink is measured. Pure glucose has a GI of 100, and this is the standard against which all other foods are compared. A GI cannot be estimated by measuring the sugar content of a particular food, as GI involves measuring the blood glucose response to a real food.

> A GI cannot be estimated by measuring the sugar content of a particular food, as GI involves measuring the blood glucose response to a real food.

Prior to GI, dieticians and nutritionalists made assumptions about simple and complex carbohydrates based on their chemical structure. It was assumed that all simple sugars were rapidly absorbed into the body, unlike complex carbohydrates that were more slowly absorbed. Simple trials soon showed this theoretical approach to be wrong. For example, eating jasmine rice results in a more rapid blood glucose surge than pure glucose in water! In fact, most starches in foods such as pasta, rice and bread are absorbed very quickly, yet some sugar foods such as icecream do not result in a high GI.

GI for a particular food is calculated as follows. A volunteer subject is given 25 or 50 grams (1 or 2 ounces) of a test food and then the blood glucose levels are measured every fifteen minutes over the first hour and then every 30 minutes over the next hour. The results are plotted on a graph. The subject's response to the test food is then compared with the subject's response to 50 grams (2 ounces) of glucose. The experiment is repeated, usually three times, and the average result calculated. The average result for around ten people is then taken to be the GI for that food. This method is surprisingly accurate, as the results for a particular food are remarkably consistent around the world. Researchers have found that they can accurately predict the GI of a meal by totalling the GI of each component. In practice, this degree of accuracy is rarely needed.

A number of factors will influence a food's GI. Acids in food delay the stomach emptying, so they slow the rate of a food's digestion. Examples of this include fruit acid (citrus juice, apples, cherries), vinegar and salad dressings. Fat also slows stomach emptying, delaying the digestion of starch. But fat has about twice as many calories as carbohydrate, so a high-fat meal will lower GI but may lead to weight gain. Clearly a balance is required. A low-GI diet does not mean that the dietary fat content can be disregarded, and it is still prudent to restrict total daily fat intake to less than 30 grams (1 ounce).

Myth: The GI is the only factor which influences the way food affects blood glucose and insulin levels.
Fact: Some foods will lower the GI of the entire meal. These include acids in foods (e.g. fruit acid and vinegar), fat, fibre and high-protein foods.

Wholemeal breads have a lower GI than white breads for several reasons. Intact grains have a fibrous coat (which takes longer to digest) protecting the starchy interior. Highly refined white flour has much smaller particles than wholemeal bread. The smaller the particles, the higher the surface area, and the easier it is for digestive enzymes to attack the food. Soluble fibre found on beans and oats seem to make the food thicker and slow down the enzymes' ability to get to the starch. Cooking and/or soaking starchy food will cause the carbohydrate to swell, bursting starch granules and making them more available to the digestive system.

Foods that are mostly composed of protein and fat will have a GI close to zero. This includes most meats, eggs, most alcoholic drinks and nuts. High-fat foods may create their own problems, especially if high in saturated fats (which can damage blood vessels). A high-fat meal may not raise blood glucose much, but most of the meal will be stored in the fat cells and so lead to an increase in weight. Also, diets that are very high in protein and fat seem to aggravate insulin resistance. It is all a matter of balance.

> Foods that are mostly composed of protein and fat will have a GI close to zero. But high-fat foods will be stored in the fat cells and increase weight.

How combining food can help

A GI of 70 or more is said to be high. A low-GI result is 55 or less (I prefer to use a GI of less than 40 as low). One important implication of all this research is that you don't have to completely avoid high-GI foods. As previously discussed, jasmine rice has a particularly high GI, but it is unusual to consume jasmine rice on its own. Having meat, vegetables and fruit with the jasmine rice bring the total GI of the meal down substantially. The rice found in sushi (nori) rolls has a high GI (because it is glutinous like jasmine rice), but the vinegar used to make sushi, and the seaweed and the vegetable filling give a sushi roll a total GI around 45 to 50. Eating four or five pieces of fruit (such as apples or citrus fruit) daily has a great effect on lowering GI, giving the best blood glucose control. Some fruit such as watermelon has a high GI (72), but most fruit has a low GI, is high in fibre and contains fruit acid which delays stomach emptying.

Myth: High-GI foods are those that rate close to 100. **Fact:** The GI of glucose is 100. A GI of 70 or more is said to be high. A low-GI result is 55 or less (40 or less is better).

GI is very important and represents a valuable addition to our knowledge about diet. Tables containing the GI of different foods are widely available. In my opinion, probably the best book on the subject of GI is *The New Glucose Revolution* (see Brand-Miller, 2004). Examples of the GI ratings of some foods are given in Table 7.6.

Controlling cholesterol and triglycerides

Everybody knows that too much fat in the diet is bad for us. Fat has about twice as many calories as sugar or protein, so eating too much of it tends to make us put on weight. Cholesterol is a soft, waxy substance that has a bad reputation, but every cell in our body needs it. Cholesterol is also used as a building block to make some of our hormones such as oestrogen. We cannot survive without some cholesterol, but too much is a major risk factor for heart attack and stroke.

Cholesterol and the other fats cannot be dissolved into our bloodstream, so have to be carried by special substances called lipoproteins. The main two lipoproteins are low-density lipoprotein (LDL) and high-density lipoprotein (HDL). If there is too much LDL in our blood, then cholesterol builds up in our arteries. HDL tends to carry cholesterol away from the artery wall and so reduce the risk of heart problems.

We get our cholesterol from our diet, mostly through animal product. It is made by the liver. Usually the body makes all the

Table 7.6 Examples of GI-rated foods

High-GI foods (GI greater than 70)

Most rice (especially jasmine, calrose)	White bread
	Most pasta
Most pretzels	Parsnips

Medium-GI foods (GI between 40 and 70)

Apricots, banana, grapes, mangoes, potatoes, raisins, watermelon	Baked beans
	Basmati rice
	Chocolate, icecream
Most breakfast cereals	Most fruit juices
Some pizza	Most egg noodles
Most potato crisps	

Low-GI foods (GI less than 40)

Cherries, apples, oranges, peaches, pears, peas, plums	Lentils, chickpeas, kidney beans
	Mars bar
	Most pizza
Milk and most yoghurts	Most soy drinks

Very low-GI foods (GI less than 10)

Beef, pork, lamb	Fish, shellfish
Avocado, bokchoy, broccoli, cabbage, cauliflower, celery, cucumber, leafy vegetables	Chicken, nuts, cheese, eggs

Source: Brand-Miller (2004).

cholesterol it needs, so it doesn't need any from the diet. Exercise tends to raise the HDL cholesterol, whereas smoking lowers it.

Triglycerides are another type of fat and are comprised of three chains. Like cholesterol, triglycerides are made by the body as well as derived from the diet. The body can convert carbohydrates into triglycerides. As discussed previously, IR is associated with high blood levels of triglycerides, so a low-GI diet, exercise and the drug metformin all improve IR and tend to lower elevated triglyceride levels. The following are the main ways to lower blood triglyceride levels:

- reduce weight;
- reduce dietary fat intake;
- reduce carbohydrate intake;
- reduce or avoid alcohol intake;
- substitute fish high in omega-3 fatty acids;
- take fish oil capsules;
- increase physical activity.

Some dietary fats are good for us. For example, omega-3 fatty acids lower triglyceride levels. Oily fish such as sardines, herrings, some tuna and salmon are all high in omega-3 fatty acids. Clinical trials have shown that a diet high in fish oils or supplements, in a dose of 0.5 to 2 grams daily, has been shown to not only reduce the blood levels of triglycerides, but also to reduce cholesterol blockages in arteries, slightly lower blood pressure and reduce the risk of death from abnormal heart rhythms. Some with very high blood triglyceride levels may need high doses of fish oil to help them.

Dietary fats are mixtures of fatty acids. Saturated fatty acids have all the hydrogen atoms that they can hold and are usually solids at room temperature. They are bad for our arteries. On the other hand, monounsaturated oils have one unsaturated bond, whereas polyunsaturated oils have many unsaturated bonds. Both of these tend to lower blood cholesterol when substituted for saturated fats.

The American Heart Foundation (www.americanheart.org) has some great information about fats and heart disease, as well as some excellent links to other information sources.

The impact of raised levels of both insulin and LH on testosterone

As already discussed, around 50 per cent of those with PCOS will have raised insulin and many also have raised LH levels. Normally, both insulin and LH act on the ovary to stimulate testosterone production (see Figure 7.3). If both blood insulin and LH levels are markedly elevated then it follows that testosterone can be quite high too. High insulin levels tend to lower SHBG thus resulting in high free, bio-active testosterone levels. PCOS is a disease characterised by vicious circles.

These insulin effects can be reversed by consuming a low-GI diet, performing at least three hours of exercise a week and by using the drug metformin. These measures tend to lower raised LH levels, although the contraceptive Pill or a GnRH agonist may be more effective.

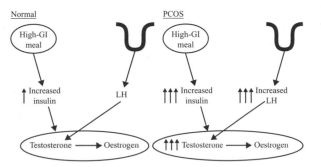

Figure 7.3 Insulin and LH both stimulate the ovary to make testosterone

Drug therapies for insulin resistance

The drug metformin is increasingly being used to treat women with PCOS. Metformin is an old drug with a long track record as a successful treatment for late-onset diabetes. It improves insulin resistance, reduces glucose uptake from the gut and aids weight loss by suppressing appetite. Currently, there is a lack of large properly conducted clinical trials, but the best information to date suggests that metformin (in a dose of 1.5 to 2 grams daily) restores ovulation in around 50 per cent of women with PCOS who are not ovulating. There is also a relative lack of information concerning foetal exposure, although some studies in South Africa, using metformin to treat pregnant diabetic women, would suggest there is not a particularly high rate of foetal abnormalities (Coetzee and Jackson, 1979 and 1986). Metformin can be very useful for the woman with PCOS and overt IR (e.g. acanthosis, raised triglycerides and/or impaired glucose tolerance) or as an adjunct to weight loss. Side-effects can include nausea and diarrhoea. Taking the tablets with food, starting with a low dose and slowly increasing the dosage over some weeks, can minimise these side-effects.

Dr Michael Costello from the Royal Hospital for Women in Sydney has reviewed the published scientific papers on the effect of metformin on women with PCOS (see Costello and Eden, 2003). He found 30 studies for the review. Twelve studies evaluated the effectiveness of metformin on the menstrual cycle. Unfortunately, nine of the studies did not have a control group. Combining the studies suggests that metformin produces regular cycles in approximately 62 per cent of women with PCOS. Most of these studies made no mention of dietary changes or an increase in exercise, so it would seem likely that combining metformin with an improved diet and exercise program might result in an even greater improvement.

Nine studies examined the effect of metformin alone on rates of ovulation. Five uncontrolled studies showed that 61 per cent of women with PCOS, who were not ovulating, began to ovulate with metformin treatment. Four randomised trials showed that a one-month trial of metformin produced an ovulation rate of 42 per cent compared with a placebo effect of 8–17 per cent. Interestingly, most studies showed that the metformin did not improve fasting insulin levels. Only four studies examined the impact of metformin treatment for women with clomiphene resistance. These were women with PCOS who were not ovulating and did not respond to clomiphene, the first-line fertility drug. Some studies found no effect, while others found that metformin was useful. Dr Costello concluded that women with PCOS having metformin for three to six months had a 60 per cent chance of restoring the cycle. Clomiphene and metformin combined for nine months gave a 66 per cent chance of ovulation and a 34 per cent chance of pregnancy. It was clear from the review that the quality of the research on metformin has been rather poor to date and that bigger and better research studies are needed.

New therapies for IR are coming through the drug development system. The most promising are the glizones (e.g. rosiglitazone). Some have been shown to improve blood profiles, but at the moment there is too little clinical research to suggest that these drugs should be offered to women with PCOS.

Patient story: Kathy, 28 years old

Kathy came to see me for a second opinion. She was having two periods a year, had mild excess body hair and had diagnosed PCOS. Her BMI was 30 (the normal range is 20–25).

Her baseline blood test results are shown in Table 7.7.

Table 7.7 Kathy's baseline blood test results

Hormone result	Kathy's results	Normal range
LH, u/L	14	2–12
FSH, u/L (mu/mL)	3 (3)	2–12 (2–12)
Prolactin, ng/ml	4	<20
TSH, mu/L	1.1	0.4–5.0
Testosterone, nmol/L (ng/dL)	4.5 (129.7)	1.5–2.6 (43.2–74.9)
SHBG, nmol/L (ng/dL)	22 (0.63)	20–120 (0.58–3.46)
DHEAS, umol/L (ng/mL)	7 (2579.2)	<11 (4053.1)
17-hydroxyprogesterone, nmol/L (g/L)	4 (1.3)	<6 (2)
Glucose, mmol/L (mg/dL)	4.7 (84.7)	3.4–5.4 (61.3–97.3)
Fasting insulin, mu/L	21	<12
Cholesterol, mmol/L (mg/dL)	4.5 (173.7)	<5.5 (<212.4)
Triglycerides, mmol/L (mg/dL)	1.8 (159.3)	<2.0 (<177)

Kathy tried the Diane-35 contraceptive Pill as a treatment for her excess hair problem. However, when her lipid levels were checked again, her triglyceride levels had risen to 4.5 mmol/L or 398.2 mg/dL (normal is <2 mmol/L or 177 mg/dL). I explained to Kathy that the oestrogen component of the Pill can raise triglyceride levels in vulnerable women and that she really needed to come off the Pill. She was sexually active, so I suggested she use barrier methods of contraception while we sorted out her hormone problems. I told her about the low-GI diet and suggested that she try metformin. I asked her to start with half a metformin 500 milligram tablet (i.e. 250 milligrams) twice daily with food. Every two to four weeks she could increase the dosage if she didn't have any side-effects, up to a maximum of two tablets twice daily. I also asked her to exercise for at least three hours a week. Over the next six months, her menstrual cycle became monthly, she lost 10 kilograms (22 pounds) in weight and her triglyceride levels fell to 0.8 mmol/L (70.8 mg/dL).

Kathy had read about Implanon, an injectible contraceptive. It does not contain oestrogen and if her triglycerides went up then the device could be removed. When I remeasured her lipids six months after inserting Implanon, her triglycerides were still well within the normal range (1.0 mmol/L or 88.5 mg/dL). Kathy had lost another 3 kilograms (6 pounds) in weight, so I suggested she stop the metformin therapy. She continued to have light monthly periods and her lipid profile remained normal.

Patient story: Jenny, 37 years old
Jenny had PCOS and a strong family history of diabetes. She had managed to keep her weight down with a low-fat diet—her BMI was 23 (normal is 20–25). She also had an active exercise program. Jenny was having about six menstrual periods per year. Her initial hormone profile is shown in Table 7.8.

Table 7.8 Jenny's initial hormone results

Hormone result	Jenny's results	Normal range
LH, u/L	9	2–12
FSH, u/L (mu/mL)	4 (4)	2–12 (2–12)
Prolactin, ng/mL	6	<20
TSH, mu/L	1.9	0.4–5.0
Testosterone, nmol/L (ng/dL)	3.2 (92.2)	1.5–2.6 (43.2–74.9)
SHBG, nmol/L (ng/dL)	40 (1.15)	20–120 (0.58–3.46)
DHEAS, umol/L (ng/mL)	7 (2579.2)	<11 (4053.1)
17-hydroxyprogesterone, nmol/L (g/L)	3 (1)	<6 (2)
Glucose, mmol/L (mg/dL)	4.1 (73.9)	3.4–5.4 (61.3–97.3)
Fasting insulin, mu/L	12	<12
Cholesterol, mmol/L (mg/dL)	4.1 (158.3)	<5.5 (<212.4)
Triglycerides, mmol/L (mg/dL)	1.5 (132.7)	<2.0 (<177)

The results of her GTT are shown in Table 7.9.

Table 7.9 Jenny's GTT results

Result	Fasting	One hour	Two hours
Blood glucose, mmol/L (mg/dL)	4.1 (73.9)	8.4 (151.4)	6.7 (120.7)
Blood insulin (mu/L)	12	154	250

The GTT results showed she was non-diabetic, but were consistent with IR. Her blood glucose response to the oral glucose load was normal. Her fasting blood insulin level was in the upper limit of normal but continued to rise even two hours after the oral glucose load.

I suggested to Jenny that she should read a book on the low-GI diet and blend the low-fat and low-GI approaches into her diet. I encouraged her to continue with her active exercise program. I told Jenny that a low-GI diet and exercise program had been shown in clinical trials to reduce the risk of diabetes by 60 per cent and that metformin reduced the risk of diabetes by 30 per cent. As three of Jenny's family had already developed late-onset diabetes, she was keen to try metformin.

What surgical procedures are available for weight loss?

Weight loss is important for those with IR. Those who have a BMI greater than 40 have about twice the risk of early death compared with a person of normal BMI (20 to 25). They are also at increased risk of heart disease, diabetes, sleep apnoea and arthritis. Those with sleep apnoea stop breathing at certain times while they are asleep. This condition is associated with tiredness and an increased risk of heart disease. If you have PCOS and a BMI more than 40, then you may find it harder to conceive naturally or with fertility drugs. Many struggle with diets and so in the past ten to twenty years there has been increasing interest in weight-loss surgery. Broadly, there are currently two main types of weight-loss operation being performed: small bowel bypass surgery and laparoscopic stomach banding.

The small bowel bypass operation

A small bowel bypass is usually done through an abdominal incision, but there is increasing interest in performing the operation through a laparoscope. There are three steps involved in the operation. First, a new small stomach pouch is made from the original stomach. Typically, the new pouch holds only about 40 millilitres (1.35 fluid ounces) of fluid and so holds a smaller amount of food and produces a feeling of fullness with relatively little food. Second, a loop of small bowel called the 'Roux limb' is joined to the new smaller stomach. Lastly, the segment of small bowel that remains is carrying fluids from the stomach, gallbladder and pancreas and this is rejoined to the small bowel.

Post-operatively, food travels down the gullet to the new small stomach and then into the Roux limb where some water and carbohydrate are absorbed but not much else. Once the food comes to the portion of the small bowel where the pancreatic juices and bile are present, further digestion can occur. In effect, this operation achieves two things: the stomach is much smaller and the absorptive capacity of the first part of the small bowel has been lost, resulting in malabsorption of many nutrients. The loss of fat and carbohydrate results in massive weight loss, but after the operation vitamin and mineral supplements are usually needed indefinitely. Some patients also have diarrhoea. It is possible to lose 30–90 per cent of the excess weight with this type of operation. But bear in mind that this is major surgery, with all its attendant risks.

The laparoscopic adjustable gastric band operation

The second, and more popular, operation involves making only the stomach smaller. In previous years, staples were used to reduce the stomach size, but the most popular operation now is the laparoscopic adjustable gastric band. The procedure is performed under a general anaesthetic using keyhole surgery. The band is placed around the upper part of the stomach, creating a small pouch on top of the band. A piece of tubing connects the band to a reservoir that is placed under the skin on the abdominal wall. Usually an x-ray is performed to check the placement of the device and then the patient is sent home, usually on the second post-operative day.

For a month after the operation, fluids only are permitted. This allows the band to fix itself to the stomach. If food is taken at this stage, vomiting can occur or the band could slip, causing a partial obstruction. Food is allowed during the second month but the change is made gradually to avoid vomiting. Band adjustments can be made at the time. Small amounts of saline are injected into the reservoir to inflate the band. Depending on the result or problems such as vomiting, saline can be added or removed simply. By the third month, most people are having five small meals per day. Most lose about two-thirds of their excess weight over one to two years. The adjustable laparoscopic gastric band operation is a less complicated and safer operation than the intestinal bypass surgery. Also, the laparoscopic band can be removed if there is a problem. Both operations require ongoing dietary monitoring.

Summary

Insulin resistance is probably an important factor for about half of those women with PCOS. The risk of having IR is highest in those with very irregular periods (say, one to two a year). There is still much debate over the best test to detect it. I believe the minimum tests that should be performed are fasting blood cholesterol and triglycerides (looking for high levels of triglycerides) as well as fasting insulin and blood glucose. A fasting insulin level greater than 12 mu/L is suggestive of IR. Fasting blood glucose greater than 7 mmol/L (126.1 mg/dL) is suggestive of diabetes. Probably the best current test for glucose intolerance is a GTT, paying particular attention to the two-hour result. A markedly elevated one- or two-hour insulin level (>60) is highly suggestive of IR; a two-hour blood glucose level more than 11 mmol/L (198.2 mg/dL) is diagnostic of diabetes. Some with IR have low blood glucose levels two to four hours after a meal, and so may need a four-hour GTT to pick up the problem.

A low-GI diet is healthy for everyone, so I tend to recommend it for all my patients. Clinical trials have shown that a low-GI diet and exercise can protect against the development of late-onset diabetes. Such an approach is likely to improve the cycle and metabolic abnormalities of PCOS. Fish oil is also useful, particularly for those with raised triglyceride levels. In selected cases, drug therapy with metformin may be indicated. Weight loss is important to prevent or control IR. For some, weight loss surgery can be very helpful.

Frequently asked questions

My weight loss diet isn't working. What can I do?

See your doctor. It is worth having a medical history taken, as well as a physical examination and perhaps a hormone check. Cortisone excess, an under-active thyroid and possible IR can aggravate weight gain. Most dieticians recommend a low-fat, low-GI diet, consuming about half your diet as carbohydrates, 30 per cent as protein and 20 per cent as fat. However, most of my patients have found it hard to lose weight with such an approach. At the other extreme, there are the high-protein diets, such as the Atkins diet, where only very small amounts of carbohydrate are permitted. These encourage weight loss, but I am concerned about the lack of fruit and vegetables in these diets. Many studies have shown that having at least five portions of fruit and vegetables daily will halve the risk of the common cancers (breast, bowel, uterine, prostate) and heart disease. I usually recommend eating plenty of fruit, vegetables and salad, and using meat, chicken, fish or soybean as a protein source. Try to minimise the intake of breads, rice and pasta. If you are going to have some bread, then the heavier the bread the better (rye, sourdough or wholegrains are best). Basmati rice is better than the glutinous rices, such as jasmine rice. In extreme cases (e.g. where your weight is over 120 kilograms or 265 pounds), weight-loss surgery can be life-saving.

What is GI?

The glycaemic index, or GI, describes how much a particular food raises blood glucose levels. The GI of glucose (sugar) is 100. Meat, chicken, fish and nuts have a GI of zero, whereas the GI of jasmine rice is 120. Thus, if you eat a piece of meat, it will not raise blood glucose levels (or insulin levels) at all. On the other hand, a bowl of jasmine rice will raise your blood glucose and insulin levels more than a Mars bar!

Can supplements help with IR?

There is some evidence that chromium supplements may help lower IR. Fish oil capsules, usually taken as 1 gram with each meal, can often help reduce raised triglyceride levels.

8
Protecting yourself:
Potential long-term health issues

Once again, it is important to emphasise the difference between having PCO and no symptoms and having PCOS. Most of the long-term health issues seem to relate to the menstrual disorder. If you are having regular periods every three to six weeks and are found to have PCO on an ultrasound scan, then there are no particular long-term hazards. You will have the same long-term risks as a similar aged woman with 'normal' ovaries on scanning.

On the other hand, those who have PCOS—especially those having only a few periods a year—may be at increased risk of a number of health problems. The main concerns raised by most PCOS patients focus on cancer and heart risks, but there are others

If you are having regular periods every three to six weeks and are found to have PCO on an ultrasound scan, then there are no particular long-term hazards.

to consider as well. There is surprisingly little research in this area; most of the available information is based on the work of Dr Eva Dahlgren's team in Sweden (1992). Her research group has been studying a group of Swedish women who had their PCOS diagnosed in the 1950s and 1960s.

What is my risk of osteoporosis?

There is always a theoretical concern that if you are not menstruating, then you may develop osteoporosis because of a lack of oestrogen. Those with PCOS usually continue to produce significant oestrogen, but have a relative lack of progesterone. Fortunately, bones only need a small amount of oestrogen to maintain strength. Men need oestrogen for their bones too, but they have only around 100 pmol/L (27.2 pg/mL) in their bloodstream. This corresponds to the level that you make during your periods—the lowest point in the menstrual cycle.

Several researchers have performed bone density studies on those with PCOS and they seem to have normal bone strength. This is in contrast to many other causes of infrequent ovulations. Conditions such as early menopause, anorexia and hypothalamic-pituitary problems all result in very low oestrogen levels. If you have one of these problems, then you may be at increased risk of developing thin bones and fractures. This complication can be prevented with sex-hormone replacements such as the contraceptive Pill, usually in combination with an adequate dietary or supplement intake of calcium (at least 1000 milligrams a day) and vitamin D (400 to 800 units per day).

Myth: Women with PCOS have less bone strength.
Fact: Women with PCOS have normal bone strength.

What is my risk of cancer?

There doesn't seem to be any good data linking PCOS to breast or ovarian cancer. There is one population study by Dr Schildkraut and colleagues (Schildkraut et al., 1996) suggesting a small increased risk of ovarian cancer; however, taking the contraceptive Pill protected against this. This is a well-known advantage of the contraceptive Pill. Women who take the Pill for more than five years more than halve their risk of ovarian cancer. On the other hand, there have been several case reports of PCOS associated with uterine cancer—that is, cancer of the lining of the uterus. (This is different to cervical cancer, which can be detected in its pre-cancerous form by a pap smear.)

Cancer of the uterine lining, or endometrial cancer, develops high up inside the uterus and it not detected by the pap smear. It usually presents with abnormal vaginal bleeding (e.g. spotting for two to four weeks). Only 10 per cent of endometrial cancer occurs in those under 40, and most of these women will have PCOS. In a recent review of PCOS, Professor Rob Norman (see Norman et al., 2004) found little evidence of an increased risk of uterine cancer. Certainly, in my 'thousand cases of PCOS' study there were no instances of uterine cancer.

The occasional case of uterine cancer associated with PCOS probably arises because of a lack of progesterone. Significant amounts of progesterone are made only after ovulation, so if you ovulate only once or twice a year, you will lack a great deal of progesterone. This allows the endometrium to thicken up, producing very heavy, infrequent periods and probably increasing the risk of uterine cancer. Either taking a contraceptive Pill or using progestin tablets (e.g. Norethisterone) for ten to fourteen days every month or two can prevent this complication. There are many studies showing that the contraceptive Pill lowers the risk of uterine cancer. The longer you take it, the lower the risk.

My research group has performed studies with 'natural' progesterone cream and found that the usual doses (1–3 per cent progesterone cream) are not strong enough to prevent pre-cancerous changes in the endometrium (Wren et al., 2000; Wren et al., 2003). In some countries, natural progesterone is available as 'micronised progesterone' in capsules. This product can certainly be used to keep the uterine lining healthy. The Mirena device contains the progestin levonorgestrel, and so effectively reduces the risk of uterine cancer and substantially reduces menstrual loss.

What is my risk of heart and blood vessel disease, and diabetes?

Many women with PCOS will also be insulin resistant and significantly overweight. This puts them at greater risk of heart disease. Some will have the so-called 'metabolic syndrome', or Syndrome X—symptoms include abdominal fatness, high cholesterol and triglycerides, high blood pressure and IR. Even if you are thin and have PCOS, you might have significant heart risk factors, such as abnormal blood fats and insulin resistance. At the moment there is a lack of solid evidence that PCOS itself increases the risk of heart and blood vessel disease. For example, one British study followed up a group of women diagnosed with PCOS between 1930 and 1979 (Pierpoint et al., 1998). It failed to show an increased risk of heart disease. Nevertheless, heart risk factors should be taken very seriously. I always check the blood fat levels of my patients, even the younger ones, as it is not unusual to find a fourteen year old with very high cholesterol or triglyceride levels.

There is no doubt that insulin resistance, the metabolic syndrome and having previously had gestational diabetes are major risk factors for developing type 2 diabetes. However, lifestyle changes can dramatically improve this situation. One large study by Dr Knowler (see Knowler et al., 2002 or www.cdc.gov.diabetes) examined those who had at least two close relatives with diabetes. All the subjects were overweight. They didn't target women with PCOS, but the results appear to be relevant for those who have

PCOS and IR. A low-GI diet and at least 30 minutes a day of exercise five days a week was found to reduce the risk of developing diabetes by 58 per cent. The drug metformin was also found to reduce the risk of developing diabetes by 31 per cent. There are many ways to minimise heart risk problems, including:

- not smoking;
- eating a low-GI, low-fat diet;
- eating at least five portions of fruit and vegetables daily;
- consuming fish or fish oils;
- getting at least three hours a week of exercise—the more vigorous the better;
- taking cholesterol-lowering and/or blood pressure drugs if needed;
- taking metformin if needed;
- controlling high blood pressure and high blood fat levels.

Summary

Women with PCOS who have an irregular cycle, such as one to two periods a year, may be at slightly increased risk of uterine cancer. Taking either a contraceptive Pill or cycles of a progestin, or being fitted with a Mirena device, could prevent this. Women with PCOS do not seem to be at increased risk of osteoporosis. However, many with PCOS do have significant heart and diabetes risk factors. A low-fat, low-GI diet combined with a sensible exercise program is recommended. If necessary, high blood pressure and high blood fat levels should be controlled with drug therapies.

Frequently asked questions

I read somewhere that women with PCO syndrome are at increased risk of osteoporosis. Is that true?

No. Women with anorexia, prolactin problems, early menopause or hypothalamic-pituitary problems may be at increased risk of osteoporosis, but not women with PCOS.

Is PCOS associated with an increased risk of cancer?

There is some mild evidence of a slightly increased risk of cancer of the uterine lining. This is reduced substantially by taking the contraceptive Pill or cycles of a progestin. The evidence concerning breast cancer and PCOS is conflicting—some studies show a slightly increased risk of breast cancer, while others show the opposite. There appears to be no good evidence of an increased risk of ovarian cancer amongst those with PCOS.

I have PCOS. What can I do to lower my risk of heart disease and diabetes?

A low-fat, low-GI diet and at least three hours a week of exercise have been shown to reduce the risk of diabetes by around 70 per cent. Avoid smoking completely. It is a good idea to have your blood pressure checked and a blood test every year or so to check your fasting cholesterol, triglyceride, glucose and perhaps insulin levels. Some women may also need medical treatments for high blood pressure, cholesterol or sugar problems.

9
Tapping into the future:
Potential new treatments

The polycystic ovary is an enigma. In some aspects it is simply a variation on normal. After all, a quarter of the female population have ovaries that look polycystic and about seven in 100 have PCOS. Clearly, there is a spectrum which ranges from regularly ovulating women with PCO and clear skin to those who have the full-blown severe PCOS with absent menstruation, severe excess body hair and insulin resistance. All medical disorders are like this. The majority with the condition have it mildly, and only a few have the severe form of the disease.

The problems associated with PCOS have been noted for decades. The management of the clinical manifestations is fairly straightforward. As discussed in previous chapters, medical research has come up with effective treatments for the skin problems of excess hair and acne, as well as ways of managing the menstrual and fertility problems. But so many questions remain. One of the biggest is why the polycystic ovary looks the way it does. Why do the follicles line up around the periphery of the ovary in a so-called 'pearl-necklace' pattern? Why is the internal part of the ovary, the stroma, enlarged? The short answer is that we simply do not know. This is just one of the many perplexing questions future research will have to answer.

What will research unveil?

There is an amazing lack of information about the best dietary approach to managing PCOS. The GI diet makes a lot of sense, but at the time of writing this book there are no studies comparing a low-GI diet with simple weight-loss or other types of diet such as a low-fat diet, vegetarianism or a high-protein diet. Considering the significant impact of body weight and diet on this condition, research into this area which compares different lifestyles and their impact on PCOS could be most enlightening. Many studies have shown that as little as 4–5 kilograms (9–11 pounds) of weight loss can often restore the cycle for an overweight woman with PCOS— but we still don't know which dietary approach is best.

There is also very little, if any, information on the impact of weight-loss surgery on the symptoms of PCOS. A number of my patients have obtained an excellent result after weight-loss surgery. They have lost considerable amounts of weight, their insulin resistance has improved and they have started to ovulate again. But there is a lack of scientific study in this area.

There is currently a lot of research taking place in the area of genetics. Microarrays are miniature chips that permit the screening of thousands and thousands of genes. This type of research is greatly simplifying the search for genes that impact on ovarian function, the insulin resistance story and PCOS. This technology allows the researcher to study the impact of multiple genes on human conditions. As I discussed earlier in Chapter 3, our 'twin study' seemed to suggest there probably isn't one 'PCO gene', although if there is a single gene then it probably lies on the X chromosome. It is more likely that several genes may act together to predispose a particular woman to the development of PCOS and these genes might interact with certain, as yet unidentified, environmental factors. Family or twin studies using microarray technology are likely to help clarify this area.

Based on current technology, it seems that just over half of those with PCOS have some evidence of insulin resistance (IR). There is still considerable debate over the exact definition of IR, what causes it and how to diagnose it. Some experts recommend using fasting insulin-to-blood glucose ratios, while others measure the blood glucose and insulin response to an oral sugar load. Currently, I prefer the latter test, but there are few studies comparing different tests. There is also argument over what causes IR. Most of those who have IR have functional blood insulin and insulin receptors, so something seems to be wrong with the target cells. Most of the problem of IR resides in the liver, muscle and fat, yet other tissues such as the ovaries remain normally sensitive to insulin. Why?

We desperately need more clinical studies into the best ways to prevent diabetes and heart disease. One large study has already been completed examining people who have at least two family members with diabetes (Knowler et al., 2002). A low-GI diet and exercise lowered diabetes risk by 58 per cent. But there are few—if any—decent, large studies of women with PCOS examining different treatment regimens over many years to find out the impact of these treatments on the risk of heart disease or diabetes.

We are fortunate indeed to have so many successful fertility treatments for women with PCOS. As discussed, weight loss, low-GI diets, metformin, clomiphene, FSH therapy and laparoscopic ovarian diathermy all improve fertility. But a few questions remain. Large placebo-controlled trials are needed to precisely study the effect of metformin on fertility. We especially need information on its safety and impact on the miscarriage rate. We still don't understand why some women with PCOS have an increased risk of miscarriage. However, weight loss, FSH thereapy and laparoscopic surgery seem to induce ovulation with the lowest miscarriage rate.

What new medical breakthroughs are likely?

The skin and the prostate share similar hormonal systems. As I discussed in Chapter 4, CPA is used to treat prostate cancer and severe hirsutism in women. With the increasing interest in hormonal therapies for prostate cancer, it is very likely that we will find novel treatments for hirsutism and acne in women. A pure anti-androgen that only has a skin effect would be clinically useful. Current anti-androgens such as CPA and spironolactone can upset the menstrual cycle, for example.

There are two other male hormone blockers available at the moment, but neither product is currently approved for use in women. Flutamine is a pure androgen blocker. It is approved for treating prostate cancer, but not yet approved (at least in Australia) for treating male hormone problems in women. Clinical trials have shown that it is an effective treatment for excess body hair. Side-effects include dry skin, loss of libido, irregular periods and nausea. Occasionally, it can also affect the liver.

Finasteride inhibits 5α-reductase and has been shown to reduce hirsutism with minimal side-effects. It is used for male-pattern baldness, and may be indicated for benign enlargement of the prostate.

What is your final summary?

As a specialist in women's hormone problems, I have seen many women with PCOS. Countless women with PCO are scared that they are infertile or will get cancer, or simply that their ovaries are 'full of cysts'. This condition seems to be afflicted by numerous urban myths. Polycystic ovaries are common, affecting about one in four women. Around half will have a skin problem such as excess body hair or acne, but most will have fairly regular periods. Medically speaking, it is normal for the menstrual periods to come every three to eight weeks. Most will have about a 28-day cycle, but by no means all. Also, polycystic ovaries do not cause pain.

The term PCOS should be reserved for those who have two of the following three symptoms:

- fewer than six periods per year;
- clinical (acne, hirsutism) and/or blood test evidence of raised androgens;
- polycystic ovaries.

The usual story is that the woman's menstrual cycle was fairly regular until she gained weight. As her weight increased, she found that her cycle lengthened. Those on a contraceptive Pill continue to have regular periods because the Pill produces an 'artificial cycle'. I have seen many who had regular periods, went on the Pill for some years, gained weight during that time and then found that their periods were very irregular when they came off the Pill. Nearly always, I find that they have PCOS and that weight gain was the trigger. Weight gain raises blood insulin levels, and high insulin levels in turn stimulate the ovaries to make more testosterone. High insulin levels also lower blood SHBG levels. These combine to cause free, bioactive testosterone levels to rise, thus lengthening the cycle and aggravating any tendency to excess body hair or acne.

Those who have irregular periods and scan evidence of PCO should be investigated further. The minimum blood work-up should include measuring blood levels of LH, FSH, Prolactin, TSH, testosterone, SHBG, DHEAS, 17-hydroxyprogesterone, lipids, glucose and insulin. It is not unusual to find scan PCO and another cause of the menstrual irregularity.

The role of diet has been greatly clarified over the last decade. I noted twenty years ago that many of my very overweight patients (weighing more than 140 kilograms or 308 pounds) with PCOS would start ovulating as soon as they started a weight-loss diet—well before they had lost any significant weight. The glycaemic index (GI) story explains why. Who would have imagined that a bowl of jasmine rice would provoke a greater blood glucose response than a drink of pure sugar? Over the past decade, nutritionists have promoted a low-fat diet for weight loss and long-term health. We were told to eat rice, pasta and bread because they are low-fat foods. Unfortunately, these foods are usually high-GI foods and consuming them produces high blood glucose and insulin responses. The insulin surges stimulate more testosterone and also cause the body to store energy in fat, rather than burning it. Three or four hours a week of exercise can halve insulin resistance in many people.

High-protein diets have also been in vogue. These certainly promote weight loss, but most of them greatly restrict fruit and vegetables. High-protein diets tend to aggravate the IR problem. Also, numerous population studies have shown that eating at least five portions of fruit and vegetables per day roughly halves the risk of four common cancers (breast, bowel, prostate and uterus) as well as heart disease. Most fruit and vegetables are low GI (but not all).

In conclusion, most of the time PCO represents a variation on normal. Those with PCO syndrome, and in particular those having fewer than six periods a year, are at increased risk of IR, diabetes and menstrual problems. However, some modest diet changes and exercise can dramatically improve their metabolic state. Many with excess body hair or acne suffer needlessly. Effective, simple and safe medical therapies are available, so these devastating skin problems can be treated. A diagnosis of PCOS should not provoke fear. I hope that I have convinced you that there is plenty of help available.

Glossary and abbreviations

<   Less than.

>   More than.

5α-reductase   The skin enzyme that converts testosterone into the very potent androgen, di-hydrotestosterone.

17-hydroxyprogesterone   A hormone made by both the ovaries and the adrenals. Blood levels of this hormone are raised in cases of CAH (see below).

Acanthosis nigricans   A dark, velvety skin condition found usually on the back of the neck or the armpits. It is strongly associated with IR.

ACTH   Adrenocorticotropin. The pituitary hormone that stimulates the adrenal glands.

Adenoma   A lump.

Adrenal gland   Hormone-producing organ sitting on top of each kidney. The adrenals make many hormones, including cortisone, androgens and adrenaline.

Adrenarche   The part of puberty in a girl that is responsible for armpit and pubic hair development. The trigger is a surge of the hormone DHEA from the adrenal glands.

AG   Androstanediol glucuronide. This hormone is produced in skin by the enzyme 5α-reductase.

Amenorrhoea   Absent periods. Usually taken as fewer than two periods a year.

Anaemia   Low red blood cell count.

Androgens   Male hormones; women convert some of their androgen into oestrogen.

Anti-androgen   Male hormone blocker.

Aromatase   The enzyme that converts androgens into oestrogens.

BBTc   Basal body temperature chart.

BMD   Bone mineral density. The main test for osteoporosis.

CAH   Congential adrenal hyperplasia. An inherited condition, where the adrenals over-produce androgens and other hormones.

Carbohydrates   Long chains of sugars.

Cervix   Neck of the uterus.

Chromosomes   These carry our genetic material. We humans have 46 chromosomes, 23 from our mother and 23 from our father.

Climacteric   The period of one to five years leading up to the menopause; *see also* Perimenopause.

Control group   A group of subjects used as a comparison with the study subjects.

Cortisone   A hormone made by the adrenal glands.

CPA   Cyproterone acetate. A progestin that is also an androgen blocker.

Cushings disease   In this condition, the adrenals over-produce cortisone.

Cyst   A fluid-filled structure more than 30 millimetres (1.18 inches) in size.

Day 1   The first day of menstrual bleeding.

DHEA   Dehydroepiandrosterone, an adrenal androgen.

DHEAS   Dehydroepiandrosterone sulphate. The most abundant hormone in the bloodstream. The sulphate molecule makes the fat-soluble DHEA into a water-soluble form, DHEAS, which is then able to be dissolved in the bloodstream.

DHT   Dihydrotestosterone. This potent androgen is made in the skin.

Embryo transfer (ET)   The process of transferring the fertilised egg into the uterus via the cervix.

Endocrine   Hormonal. Specifically, it means that the hormone is released directly into the bloodstream.

Endometriosis   A disease where tissue that resembles the uterine lining is growing outside the uterus. Symptoms include pelvic pain, irregular bleeding and sometimes difficulty conceiving.

Endometrium   Internal lining of the uterus. This is the part that bleeds each month.

Epidemiology   The study of disease in relation to populations.

FAI   Free androgen index. $FAI = \dfrac{\text{total testosterone} \times 100}{\text{SHBG}}$. The FAI is a measure of free testosterone.

Fibroids   Balls of muscle and fibre that enlarge the uterus, sometimes causing heavy periods and pain.

Follicle   A fluid-filled structure in the ovary less than 30 millimetres in diameter.

Free testosterone   The biologically active portion of testosterone.

FSH   Follicle stimulating hormone. The pituitary hormone which stimulates the follicle to grow and produce sex hormones like oestrogen.

fT3   Free triiodothyronine. The biologically active portion of the most potent thyroid hormone.

fT4   Free thyroxine. The biologically active portion of the main thyroid hormone.

Glycaemic index (GI)   This refers to how quickly a food raises blood glucose.

Glycaemic load (GL)   The glycaemic load predicts how much a particular food will raise blood glucose. Glycaemic load is the GI of a food multiplied by the amount of carbohydrate in the food divided by 100 (GL = [GI $\times$ grams] / 100).

GnRH   Gonadotropin releasing hormone. GnRH is normally released in 90-minute pulses from the cyclic centre. This in turn triggers the pituitary to release LH and FSH. GnRH is the pulse of the cyclic centre.

Goitre   Enlarged thyroid gland.

Gut flora   Friendly bowel germs that help us digest our food.

HCG   Human chorionic gonadotrophin. This is the 'pregnancy hormone'. It has actions very similar to LH and so is often used as a source of LH activity for ovulation induction.

Heritability index (HI)   If HI approaches 1.0 then genetic factors are likely. If HI approaches 0, then non-genetic factors are more likely to be important.

Hg   Mercury.

HGH   Human growth hormone.

Hirsutism   Excess body hair.

HMG   Human menopausal gonadotrophins. A source of FSH derived from the urine of menopausal women.

Hormone   Chemical messengers which target specific cells.

Hormone receptors   Specialised proteins that permit hormones to enter a cell and then act in the cell. Each hormone has a specific receptor(s). It is a bit like a lock and key: the hormone is the key and the receptor is the lock.

HRT   Hormone replacement therapy. Refers to oestrogen and progestin therapy given to women who are not making enough sex hormones.

Hyperthyroidism   Over-active thyroid gland.

Hypothalamus   A small area of the brain on top of the pituitary. The hypothalmus regulates many automatic bodily functions such as temperature control.

Hypothyroidism   Under-active thyroid gland.

Hysterectomy   Removal of the uterus.

Insulin   A hormone made by the pancreas gland and released into the bloodstream in response to rising blood glucose levels. Insulin lowers blood glucose and helps cells use glucose as a fuel.

In-vitro fertilisation (IVF)   Fertilisation of an egg and sperm outside the body.

IR   Insulin resistance.

IUD   Intrauterine device.

IVF   In-vitro fertilisation.

Laparoscopy   A type of keyhole surgery.

LAVH   Laparoscopic-assisted vaginal hysterectomy. Keyhole surgery is used to free the uterus from above, then the uterus is removed through the vagina.

LG   Levonorgestrel, a progestin.

LH   Luteinising hormone. A pituitary hormone that works in tandem with FSH to stimulate ovulation and the ovarian production of sex hormones (mostly androgens).

Macrodenoma   Solid lump (>10 millimetres or 0.39 inches).

Mastalgia   Breast pain.

Menarche   First menstrual period.

Menopause   Last spontaneous menstrual period. Ovarian failure: the ovaries have run out of eggs.

Metabolic syndrome   Three out of the following five need to be present: waist measurement >88 centimetres (35 inches); raised blood triglycerides; raised blood HDL-c; raised blood pressure; abnormal GTT (impaired glucose tolerance).

Microadenoma   Small solid lump (<10 millimetres or 0.39 inches).

Ml   Millilitres (one thousandth of a litre).

Mm   Millimetres (one thousandth of a metre).

Mmol/l   Millimoles per litre.

Monosaccharide   One sugar molecule.

MPA   Medroxyprogesterone acetate. A synthetic progestin.

Mu/l   Microunit per litre.

Multicystic ovaries   The normal appearance of the ovaries around puberty.

Ng/ml   Nanograms per millilitre.

Nmol/l   Nanomoles per litre.

OCP   Oral contraceptive Pill.

Oestradiol   The main, and the most potent, human oestrogen.

Oestrogen   The main female hormone. It is mostly produced by the ovaries, but significant amounts are also made by fat, and during pregnancy by the placenta.

Oligomenorrhoea   Infrequent periods: usually taken as two to ten periods a year.

Oocyte   Egg or ovum.

Osteoporosis   Low bone density (a T score <2.5 on bone density testing) that can lead to fractures.

Ovarian diathermy   An operation, usually performed as keyhole surgery, where the ovaries are burned. Somehow this can restore ovulation in many women with PCOS.

Ovulation   The process which involves the growth of a follicle and release of the egg.

Ovum donation (OD)   Egg donation.

PCO   Polycystic ovaries. There is a 'pearl-necklace' pattern of more than twelve small follicles arranged around the periphery of the ovary. The PCO usually have a volume of more than 10 millilitres or 0.3 fluid ounces (a teaspoon holds about 5 millilitres or 0.2 fluid ounces of water).

PCOS   Polycystic ovary syndrome. Two of the following three need to be present: fewer than six periods a year; clinical or blood test evidence of raised androgens; PCO present.

Perimenopause   The time leading up to the last period, usually associated with some menstrual irregularity and episodic oestrogen deficiency symptoms; *see also* Climacteric.

Phytoestrogens   Plant oestrogens; these are very weak oestrogens.

Pill, the   The contraceptive Pill.

Pituitary   A small gland that sits at the base of the brain, behind the nose.

PMT   Premenstrual tension.

Polysaccharides   Chains of many sugar molecules.

Postmenopausal   The phase of life after the menopause.

Progesterone   A female hormone which, broadly speaking, has an anti-oestrogen action. It is usually made by the ovary after ovulation and by the placenta during pregnancy.

Progestin   A synthetic hormone with progesterone actions (e.g. Norethisterone). Progestins lighten the periods and protect the uterus against cancer.

Prolactin   The pituitary hormone that stimulates breast milk production.

RCT   Randomised controlled trial. This is where half the subjects receive the active treatment and the other half are given a dummy treatment.

rhCG   Recombinant hCG.

rLH   Recombinant LH.

SHBG   Sex hormone binding globulin. SHBG is a protein made by the liver, which binds mostly testosterone, but also oestrogens to a lesser extent. Hormone that is bound to SHBG is thought to be biologically inactive—only the unbound or 'free' hormone is active.

Sheehan's syndrome   Pituitary failure following shock, usually blood loss.

Study population   A group of subjects under investigation.

T3   Triiodothyronine. The most potent thyroid hormone.

T4   Thyroxine. One of the thyroid hormones.

Testosterone   The main male hormone (in both sexes).

TSH   Thyroid stimulating hormone. The pituitary hormone that regulates the thyroid.

Ultrasound   An imaging technique that uses soundwaves.

U/L   Units per litre.

Umol/l   Micromoles per litre.

Uterus   Womb; muscular organ which carries the foetus.

References and further reading

Adams, J., Polson, D.W. and Franks, S. (1986). Prevalence of polycystic ovaries in women with anovulation and idiopathic hirsutism. *British Medical Journal*, 293: 355–9. *(One of the first papers showing that polycystic ovaries are really common, especially amongst women with excess body hair.)*

Amirika, H., Savog-Moore, R.T., Sandareson, A.S. and Moghissi, K.S. (1986). Effects of androgens on the ovary. *Fertility and Sterility*, 46: 343–4.

Barman Balfour, J.A. and McClellan, K. (2001). Topical eflornithine. *American Journal of Clinical Dermatology*, 2: 197–201. *(A very good review on this topical hirsutism treatment.)*

Bone, Kerry (2000). *Principles and Practice of Phytotherapy: Modern Herbal Medicines*, Churchill Livingstone, Edinburgh and New York. *(An extremely useful resource on herbals. One of the best herbal textbooks in the world.)*

Brand-Miller, J. (2004). *The New Glucose Revolution*. 4th edn. Hodder Headline, Sydney. *(This is an excellent book on GI and a very effective dietary approach to PCOS.)*

Bunker, C.B., Newton, J.A., Kilborn, J. et al. (1989). Most women with acne have polycystic ovaries. *British Journal of Dermatology*, 121: 675–80.

Clark, A.M., Thornley B. and Tomlinson, L. (1998). Weight loss in obese infertile women results in improvement in reproductive outcomes for all forms of fertility treatment. *Human Reproduction*, 13: 1502–8.

Clayton, R.N., Ogden, V., Hodgkinson, J. et al. (1992). How common are polycystic ovaries in normal women and what is their significance for the fertility of the population? *Clinical Endocrinology*, 37: 127–34. *(Shows that polycystic ovaries are commonly found amongst normal women.)*

Clifford, K., Rai, R., Watson, H., Franks, S. and Regan, L. (1996). Does suppressing LH secretion reduce the miscarriage rate? Results of a randomised controlled trial. *British Medical Journal*, 312: 1508–11. *(This is one of the few properly conducted clinical trials on treatments for miscarriage amongst women with PCOS. It compared a treatment that corrected one of the major hormone abnormalities found amongst women with PCOS, namely high blood LH levels. However, the treatment made no difference to the pregnancy outcome.)*

Coetzee, E.J. and Jackson, W.P.U. (1979) Metformin in management of pregnant insulin dependent diabetes. *Diabetogia*, 16: 241–5.

——(1986). The management of non-insulin-dependent diabetes during pregnancy. *Diabetes Research and Clinical Practice*, 1: 201–87.

Cooper, H.E., Spellecy, W.N., Prem, K.A. and Cohen, W.D. (1968). Hereditary factors in the Stein Leventhal syndrome. *American Journal of Obstetrics and Gynecology*, 100: 371–87.

Costello, M.F. and Eden, J.A. (2003). A systematic review of the reproductive system effects of metformin in patients with PCO syndrome. *Fertility and Sterility*, 79(1): 1–13. *(This is an up-to-date review of the use of metformin in PCOS.)*

Dahlgren, E., Johanssan, S., Hindstedt, G., Oden, A., Jansan, P.O., Mattsan, L.A., Crona, N. and Lundbert, P.A. (1992). Women with PCOS wedge resected in 1956–65: A long-term follow-up focusing on natural history and circulating hormones. *Fertility and Sterility*, 57: 505–13.

Dale, P.O., Tambo, T., Haug, E. and Abyholm, T. (1992). PCOS: Low dose FSH administration is a safe stimulation regimen even in previous hyperesponsive patients. *Human Reproduction*, 7(8): 1085–9.

Dunaif, A. (1986). Do androgens directly regulate gonadotropin secretion in polycystic ovary syndrome? *Journal of Clinical Endocrinology and Metabolism*, 63: 215–21. *(This study indicated that the high LH found in some cases of PCOS is not due to the high levels of androgens.)*

——(1997). Insulin resistance and the polycystic ovary syndrome: Mechanisms and implications for pathogenesis. *Endocrine Review*, 18(6): 774–800. *(An excellent scientific review on insulin resistance and PCOS.)*

Eden, J.A. (1988). Which is the best test to detect the polycystic ovary? *Australian and New Zealand Journal of Obstetrics and Gynaecology*, 28: 221–4. *(This paper compares different blood tests to find the best one to diagnose PCOS syndrome.)*

——(1989). The polycystic ovary syndrome—a review. *Australian and New Zealand Journal of Obstetrics and Gynaecology*, 29: 403–16.

——(1991). The polycystic ovary syndrome presenting as resistant acne, successfully treated with cyproterone acetate. *Medical Journal of Australia*, 155: 677–80. *(This is the paper on severe acne, PCOS and Androcur quoted in Chapter 4.)*

Eden, J.A., Place, J., Carter, G.D., Jones, J., Alaghband-Zadeh, J. and Pawson, M.E. (1989a). Is the polycystic ovary a cause of infertility in ovulatory women? *Clinical Endocrinology*, 30: 77–82. *(A study of polycystic ovaries amongst women having trouble conceiving.)*

—— (1989b). The role of chronic anovulation in the polycystic ovary syndrome—normalization of sex-hormone binding globulin levels after clomiphene induced ovulation. *Clinical Endocrinology*, 30: 323–32. *(This study showed that not ovulating lowers SHBG levels, and restoring ovulation with clomiphene restores SHBG levels to normal.)*

——(1989c). The diagnosis of polycystic ovaries in subfertile women. *British Journal of Obstetrics and Gynaecology*, 96: 809–15. *(A paper reviewing the diagnosis of PCOS amongst women having trouble conceiving.)*

Eden, J.A. and Warren, P. (1999). A review of 1019 consecutive cases of polycystic ovary syndrome demonstrated by ultrasound. *Australasian Radiology*, 43: 41–6. *(This is the thousand cases of PCOS paper.)*

Farquhar, C.M., Birdsall, M., Manning, P. et al. (1994). The prevalence of polycystic ovaries on ultrasound scanning in a population of randomly selected women. *Australian and New Zealand Journal of Obstetrics and Gynaecology*, 34: 67–72. *(A New Zealand paper on the rate of polycystic ovaries in a normal population.)*

Farquhar, C.M., Williamson, K., Gudex, G., Johnsan, N.P., Garland, J. and Sadler, L. (2002). A randomised controlled trial of laparoscopic ovarian diathermy versus gonadotropin therapy for women with clomiphene citrate-resistant PCOS. *Fertility and Sterility*, 78(2): 404–11.

Ferriman, D. and Purdie, A.W. (1979). The inheritance of PCO and the possible relationship to premature balding. *Clinical Endocrinology*, 11: 771–83.

Givens, J.R. (1988). Familial polycystic ovarian disease. *Endocrinology and Metabolism Clinics of North America*, 17: 771–83.

Gjonnaess, H. (1989). The course and outcome of pregnancy after ovarian electrocautery in women with polycystic ovary syndrome: The influence of body weight. *British Journal of Obstetrics and Gynaecology*, 96: 714–19. *(This is a good paper written by one of the pioneers of ovarian diathermy for PCOS.)*

———(1998). Late endocrine effects of ovarian electrocautery in women with polycystic ovary syndrome. *Fertility and Sterility*, 69(4): 697–701. *(One of the few long-term studies of the effects of ovarian diathermy. Dr Gjonnaess is one of the pioneers of this operation. In this paper he describes results in 165 women who had the operation. Most had improved blood results (lower LH and lower androgens) and more frequent ovulations. Unlike other studies, he found that these changes persisted for years after the operation. Eighteen to twenty years after the operation, 74 per cent of the women who were initially not ovulating were still ovulating.)*

Goldheizer, J.W. and Green, J.A. (1962). The polycystic ovary. I. Clinical and Histological features. *Journal of Clinical Endocrinology and Metabolism*, 72: 325–38. *(A classic PCOS paper written 40 years ago. When I first read this, I realised that things had not advanced much in 40 years.)*

Greenblatt, E. and Casper, R. (1993). Adhesion formation after laparoscopic ovarian cautery for PCOS: Lack of correlation with pregnancy rate. *Fertility and Sterility*, 60: 766–70.

Hassan, M.A.M. and Killick, S.R. (2003). Ultrasound diagnosis of polycystic ovaries in women who have no symptoms of PCOS is not associated with subfecundity or subfertility. *Fertility and Sterility*, 80(4): 966–75.

Holte, J., Gennarelli, G., Wide, L. et al. (1998). High prevalence of polycystic ovaries and associated features in women with previous gestational diabetes mellitus. *Journal of Clinical Endocrinology and Metabolism*, 83: 1143–50. *(One of the studies showing a link between PCOS and diabetes of pregnancy.)*

Jahanfar, S. and Eden, J.A. (1993). Idiopathic hirsutism or polycystic ovary syndrome? *Australian and New Zealand Journal of Obstetrics and Gynaecology*, 33(4): 414–16. *(This study showed that most women with excess hair and regular periods have polycystic ovaries.)*

——(1995). Bulimia nervosa and polycystic ovary syndrome. *Gynecological Endocrinology*, 9: 113–17. *(A study of the link between PCOS and eating disorders.)*

——(1996). Genetic and non-genetic theories on the aetiology of polycystic ovary syndrome. *Gynecological Endocrinology*, 10: 357–64. *(A review of the causes of polycystic ovaries.)*

Jahanfar, S., Eden, J.A., Warren, P., Seppala, M. and Nguyen, T. (1995). A twin study of polycystic ovary syndrome. *Fertility and Sterility*, 63: 478–86. *(This is the twin PCOS paper.)*

Jahanfar, S., Nguyen, T., Eden, J.A., Wang, X.L. and Wilcen, D.E.L. (1997). A twin study of polycystic ovary syndrome and lipids. *Gynecological Endocrinology*, 11(2): 111–18. *(A twin study of polycystic ovaries and lipids.)*

Jenkins, D.J., Wolever, T.M. and Taylor, R.H. (1981). Glycemic index of food: A physiological basis for carbohydrate exchange. *American Journal of Clinical Nutrition*, 34(3): 362–6.

Kahsar-Miller, M.D., Nixon, C., Boots, L.R. et al. (2001). Prevalence of polycystic ovary syndrome in first degree relatives of patients with PCOS. *Fertility and Sterility*, 75(1): 53–8. *(A recent family study of PCOS. They found that, amongst patients with PCOS, between 24 and 32 per cent of their mothers and sisters had PCOS too.)*

Kiddy, D.S., Hamilton-Fairley, D., Bush, A. et al (1992). Improvement in endocrine and ovarian function during dietary treatment of obese women with polycystic ovary syndrome. *Clinical Endocrinology*, 36: 105–11. *(One of the first papers showing that weight loss improves the blood profile and symptoms of PCOS.)*

Knowler, W.C., Barrett-Connor, E., Fowler, S.E. et al. (2002). Reduction in the incidence of type 2 diabetes with life-style intervention or metformin. *New England Journal of Medicine*, 346(6): 393–403. *(This is the important study that showed that high-risk individuals for diabetes can lower their risk with lifestyle changes or metformin.)*

Laitinen, J., Taponen, S. and Martikainen, H. (2003). Body size from birth to adulthood as a predictor of self reported PCOS. *International Journal of Obesity Related Metabolic Disorders*, 27(6): 710–15.

Liddell, H.S., Sowden, K. and Farquhar, C.M. (1997). Recurrent miscarriage: Screening for polycystic ovaries and subsequent pregnancy outcome. *Australian and New Zealand Journal of Obstetrics and Gynaecology*, 37(4): 402–6. *(A reassuring paper about miscarriage and PCOS. The 73 women in the study had each suffered more than three miscarriages and 26 of them (36 per cent) had polycystic ovaries. The miscarriage rate amongst those with polycystic ovaries was 18 per cent, which is much the same as normal.)*

Ludwig, M., Westergaard, L.G., Diedrick, K. and Andersen, C.Y. (2003). Developments in drugs for ovarian stimulation. *Best Practice Research, Clinical Obstetrics and Gynecology*, 17(2): 231–47.

Marynick, S.P., Chakmakjian, Z.H., McCaffree, D.C. and Herndan, J.H. (1983). Androgen excess in cystic acne. *New England Journal of Medicine*, 308: 981–5.

McClusky, S., Evans, C., Lacey, J.H., Pearce, J.M. and Jacobs, H. (1992). Polycystic ovary syndrome and bulimia. *Fertility and Sterility*, 55: 287–91. *(A study examining the link between PCOS and eating disorders.)*

Mills, S. and Bone, K. (2000). *Principles and Practice of Phytotherapy.* Churchill Livingstone Press, London. *(An excellent book on medicinal herbals.)*

Norman, R.J., Wu, R. and Stankiewicz, M.T. (2004). Polycystic ovary syndrome. *Medical Journal of Australia*, 180: 132–7. *(An excellent short Australian review of PCOS.)*

Pierpont, T., McKeigue, P.M. and Isaacs, A.J. (1998). Mortality of women with PCOS at long-term follow-up. *Journal of Clinical Epidemiology*, 51: 581–6.

Polson, D.W., Wadsworth, J., Adams, J. and Franks, S. (1988). Polycystic ovaries—a common finding in normal women. *The Lancet*, 16 April: 870–2. *(Probably the first study to show that polycystic ovaries are common amongst perfectly normal, healthly women.)*

Rai, R., Backos, M., Rushworth, F. and Regan, L. (2000). Polycystic ovaries and recurrent miscarriage—a reappraisal. *Human Reproduction*, 15(3): 612–15. *(The authors followed 2199 women with polycystic ovaries. They found that these women did not have an increased rate of miscarriage at all.)*

Rotterdam ESHRE/ASRM-Sponsored Consensus PCOS Workshop Group (2004). Revised 2003. Consensus on diagnostic criteria and long-term health risks related to PCOS. *Fertility and Sterility*, 81: 19–25. *(This paper contains the latest consensus definitions of PCO, PCOS and metabolic syndrome.)*

Schildkraut, J.M., Schwingl, P.J., Bastos, E., Evanoff, A. and Hughes, C. (1996). Epithelial cancer risk among women with polycystic ovary syndrome. *Obstetrics and Gynecology*, 88: 554–9.

Schulz, V., Hansel, R. and Tyler, V.E. (2001). *Rational Phytotherapy.* 4th edn. Springer Press, Berlin. *(Another excellent, science-based book on medicinal herbs.)*

Simmons, D., Walters, B.N.J., Rowan, J.A. and McIntyre, H.D. (2004). Metformin therapy and diabetes in pregnancy. *Medical Journal of Australia*, 180: 462–4.

Stein, I.F. (1956). Ultimate results of bilateral ovarian wedge resection: 25 year follow-up, 29: 181–91.

Stein, I.F. and Leventhal, M.L. (1935). Amenorrhoea associates with bilateral polycystic ovaries. *American Journal of Obstetrics and Gynecology*, 29: 181–91. *(The classic paper on polycystic ovaries.)*

Tsilchorozidou, T., Overton, C. and Conway, G. (2004). The pathophysiology of PCOS. *Clinical Endocrinology*, 60: 1–17. *(A recent review on the possible causes of PCOS.)*

Urbanek, M., Legro, R.S., Driscoll, D.A. et al. (1999). Thirty-seven candidate genes for polycystic ovary syndrome: The strongest evidence for linkage is with follistatin. *Proceedings of the National Acadamy of Sciences, USA*, 96: 8573–8. *(A good paper on likely genes involved in PCOS.)*

Venturoli, S., Porcu, E., Fabbri, R. et al. (1987). Postmenarchal evolution of endocrine and ovarian aspects in adolescents with menstrual irregularities. *Fertility and Sterility*, 48(1): 78–85. *(A classic paper showing that, contrary to popular belief, most girls who begin menstruation with irregular periods do not normalise their cycle. Most will have polycystic ovaries and continue to have irregular periods.)*

Wajchenberg, B.L., Achando, S.S., Okada, H. et al. (1986). Determination of the source of androgen overproduction by stimultaneous adrenal and ovarian venous catheterisation. Comparison with the dexamethasone suppression test. *Journal of Clinical Endocrinology and Metabolism*, 636: 1204–10. *(This study shows that the ovaries are the main source of androgen over-production.)*

Wild, S., Pierpoint, T., McKeigue, P. and Jacobs, H.S. (2000). Cardiovascular disease in women with polycystic ovary syndrome at long-term follow-up: A retrospective cohort study. *Clinical Endocrinology*, 52: 595–600. *(This study was performed by a well-respected PCO research group and found that, although women with PCOS had a high risk of heart risk factors, they did not have an increased risk of heart disease.)*

Wren, B.G., Champian, S.M. and Willettes, K. (2003). Transdermal progesterone and its effect on vasomotor symptoms, blood lipid levels, base metabolic markers, moods and quality of life for post menopausal women. *The Journal of the North American Menopause Society*, 10(1): 13–18.

Wren, B.G., McFarland, K. and Edwards, L. (2000). Effect of sequential progesterone cream on endometrium, bleeding pattern and plasms progesterone and salivary progesterone levels in post menopausal women. *Climacteric*, 3: 155–60.

Yen, S.S.C. (1980). *The Polycystic Ovary*, 12: 177–208. *Clinical Endocrinology*.

Useful websites

There is an enormous amount of information available via the internet, but a few things need to be kept in mind. Most medical websites emphasise the severe end of most disorders. Remember that the majority of people will have the condition mildly, some moderately and a few severely. PCOS is a good example. Most women who have polycystic ovaries have no symptoms at all. Most will have regular cycles, varying from three to eight weeks. Only 7 per cent will have fewer than six periods a year (part of our definition of PCOS), and only 1–2 per cent will have virtually no periods.

Always keep in mind that those with the worst problem will occupy chat rooms. Someone who has PCOS and no problems isn't going to waste her time setting up a website or a chat room. Anyone can set up a website, so don't believe everything you see. I tend to stick to websites put together by reputable bodies such as universities, government bodies or large teaching hospitals. I spent several hours trying to find a specific PCOS website that I could recommend—one that comprehensively covered all aspects of PCO syndrome. I couldn't find it. However, there are some very good sites on various aspects of PCOS.

With all this in mind, following are some of my favourite websites. I hope that you find them useful too.

www.contraceptiononline.org

This is an excellent website on contraception issues. It is suitable for health professionals and the general public. One can readily access information about the expert panel (the website contains their CVs). It covers all aspects of contraception and is constantly updated. This website even has a page where slide presentations can be downloaded in Powerpoint format. It also contains a 'frequently asked questions' section. Note that the website was sponsored by Wyeth, a large US company that makes oral contraceptive Pills, with an 'unrestricted educational grant'. This means that Wyeth gave the money to a university (Baylor College of Medicine), but had no influence over the content of the website. In other words, they gave the money, and the college put together the information.

www.menopause.org

This is the website for the North American Menopause Society. It is one of the best menopause websites in the world. It contains information of interest to the general public and to doctors.

www.mayohealth.org

The website for the Mayo Clinic in the United States (one of the most prestigious hospitals in America). It is comprehensive, covering most medical disorders including many women's health matters. It is one of the best health sites on the web.

www.nccam.nih.gov

The website for the US National Centre for Complementary and Alternative Medicine. This is the authoritative site on alternative medical matters.

www.healthywomen.org

This is a good website covering many aspects of women's health. It clearly states its editorial policy and, although it is sponsored by Johnson and Johnson and other companies, they have no editorial control.

www.nicls.com.au

This fabulous reference piece can be accessed for free, via the National Institute of Clinical Studies website. The Cochrane database can also be accessed through this site. The Cochrane group produces comprehensive reviews on medical treatments by performing a statistical technique called 'meta-analysis'. This involves collecting all the available data on a subject, weighing the evidence and mathematically blending it all together to produce a statistical review.

www.herbmed.org

One of the best free websites on herbals that I have found. It has comprehensive information on over 100 herbs with not only references, summaries and articles on all aspects of each herb, but also excellent links to other websites. I looked up garlic and found 65 clinical trials, 28 case reports and 27 records of traditional and folk usage. There were nearly 400 papers on how garlic works, about 80 papers on potential side-effects as well as information on topics such as formulations, links, interactions and contraindications. HerbMed is owned by a public charity and clearly identifies its sources of funding.

www.health.nih.gov

This is the web page for the US Department of Health. It has an easy-to-use search engine that permits quick access to reliable information on many human conditions. It also contains a number of free resources, including MEDLINE, which allows search and retrieval of most scientific papers quickly and easily.

www.healthfinder.gov

Another US government-sponsored reliable website for health. A good place to start if you are looking for good quality information on a medical condition.

www.cancer.org

The website for the American Cancer Society. An excellent resource for high-quality, reliable information on cancer.

www.hormone.org

The Hormone Foundation is the public education arm of the American Endocrine Society. I found that it carried a lot of good information on PCOS as well as some excellent links (e.g. to American Food and Drug Administration, HealthFinder, MEDLINE Plus, National Institutes of Health and the Women's Health project, to name a few).

www.americanheart.org

The American Heart Foundation has some great information about fats and heart disease, as well as some excellent links to other information sources.

www.cdc.gov/diabetes

The website for the American National Center for Chronic Disease Prevention. The diabetes link is excellent, with current up-to-date information about preventing and treating diabetes.

www.plasticsurgery.org

The website of the American Society of Plastic Surgeons. It has some excellent information about surgical methods for dealing with scarring, especially acne-induced scars.

www.aad.org

The American Academy of Dermatology's website is an excellent resource on the subject of chemical peels.

www.billings-centre.ab.ca

If you are interested in natural family planning, then this is the website for you.

Index

abdominal ultrasound 20, 29
acne 4, 16, 46, 50–3
    and contraceptive Pill 61, 63, 65, 70, 115
    dermatological approaches 59–60
    scarring 58–9
    study 51–3
adenoma 56
adenomyosis 96, 97
adrenal glands 55–6, 91–4
Androcur 49, 52
androgen 5, 9–10, 37, 38, 46, 47, 50, 56
anorexia nervosa 84
anti-inflammatory tablets 104

blood tests 23–9
blood vessel disease 177–8
body hair 2, 4, 5, 16, 38, 46–50, 55, 57–8, 61
body mass index (BMI) 42, 49, 76, 84

cancer 102, 114, 119, 174, 176–7, 179, 183
carbohydrates 157–8

cholesterol 150, 162–4, 172
clomiphene 86, 127–34, 166
congenital adrenal hyperplasia (CAH) 56, 91–4
contraception
    and PCOS 112–21
    natural family planning 121
    sterilisation 120–1
contraceptive Pill 52, 60–3, 65, 69–70, 100, 103, 105, 115–19
    and acne 61, 63, 65, 70, 115
    and cancer 176
    and fertility 118
    and PCOS 36, 37, 118–19
    health benefits 118–19
    menstrual irregularity 100, 103, 105, 119
    side-effects 116–17
contraceptives
    barrier 113–14
    injectible 119–20
    intrauterine devices 114–15
corpus luteum 6
Cushing's syndrome 95
Cyclokapron 26

Cyproterone acetate (CPA) 49, 52, 64–6,
100, 183

Dalkon shield 114
danazol 99
dehydroepiandrosterone (DHEA) 9–10
dehydroepiandrosterone sulphate
(DHEAS) 52
desogestrel 115
dexamethasone 93
diabetes 177–8
gestational 125, 142, 143–4, 177
Diane-35 61, 62, 65, 71, 115
diet 39–42, 45, 74, 126–7, 144, 148,
156–62, 172, 184–5
dihydrotestosterone (DHT) 35, 48
dydrogesterone 100

eating disorders 39, 40
eflornithine 67–8
endocrine glands 7, 8
endometrial cancer 102, 106
endometriosis 96, 97–9
endometrium 6, 97, 102
environment and PCOS 39–42
erythromycin 60
excess hair see hair; hirsutism
exercise
and diabetes 178
and ovulation 125, 126–7, 144

5α-reductase 48–9, 183
family planning, natural 121
fasting insulin level 28
fats and diet 157–9, 162–4
female foetus 39
female hormones 75
Femoden-ED 115
fertility issues 86, 110–47
and lifestyle 125
and medical treatments 126–39
and PCOS 111–13, 122, 142–5
barrier contraceptives 113–14
injectible contraception 119–20
intrauterine devices 114–15
natural family planning 121
ovulation 122–5, 134–8, 148

sterilisation 120–1
surgical treatments 140–2
fibroids 96, 97
fish oil 164, 172
flutamine 183
follicle stimulating hormone (FSH) 8,
13–14, 127, 128
therapy 86, 133, 134–9, 143
follicles 3
food and PCOS 39–42, 45, 148, 156–7
free androgen index (FAI) 28
free testosterone levels 28, 74

genetics and PCOS 32–4, 44
gestational diabetes 125, 142, 143–4, 177
glucagon 149
glycaemic index (GI) 125, 157, 158,
159–62, 163, 172, 173, 178, 184–5
gonadotropin releasing hormone
(GnRH) 13, 86, 99
Grave's disease 90

hair
body 2, 4, 5, 16, 38, 46–50, 55, 57–8,
60–1, 69–70
follicles 47, 48, 49
loss 26, 46, 54, 68, 70
removal 57–8
Hashimoto's disease 90
heart disease 177–8
hirsutism
and contraceptive Pill 60–1, 69–70
natural therapies 69
severe 46–50, 183
see also hair
homeostasis model assessment (HOMA)
152, 155
hormonal-related symptoms 5
hormonal tests 55–6
hormone replacement therapy (HRT)
88, 89, 102–3, 121
hormones 6, 7–8, 15–16
female 75
male 5, 9, 16, 17–18, 37–8, 39, 48–9,
183
sex 9–15, 53–5
human growth hormone (HGH) 6

hyperthyroidism 90
hypothalamic-pituitary problems 84–7
hypothalamus 8, 12–13
hypothyroidism 90
hysterectomy 97, 107–8

insulin 74, 148, 164–5, 172, 182, 185
insulin resistance (IR)
    and diabetes 177
    and diets 185
    blood tests 152–6
    control and prevention 156–62
    defined 149–50
    diagnosis 150–2
    drug therapies 165–9
    polycystic ovary syndrome (PCOS)
        28, 39, 43, 126, 128, 149–62, 172,
        182
intrauterine devices 106, 114–15
iron supplements 68–9
isoflavones 40
isotretinoin 51, 60

Kallman's syndrome 86

laparoscopic surgery for PCOS 140–2
laparoscopy 2, 21
levonorgestrel (LG) 106
lifestyle and fertility 125
Loette 61

male hormones 5, 9, 16, 17–18, 37–8, 39,
    48–9
Marvelon 105, 115
menarche 6
menopause 11
    premature 88–9
menstrual cycle 5, 6–15, 16, 38, 72,
    148
menstrual irregularity 5, 23, 24, 56,
    72–109
    adrenal problems 91–4
    and PCOS 73–80, 111
    and stress 81–2
    anorexia nervosa 84
    anti-inflammatory tablets 104
    contraceptive Pill 100, 103, 105, 119

control of 101–8, 165–9
    Cushing's syndrome 95
    hypothalamic-pituitary problems
        84–7
    hysterectomy 107–8
    Mirena device 106, 144
    premature menopause 88–9
    progestin 99–100, 105
    prolactin problems 82–3
    surgery, conservative 106–7
    thyroid problems 89–91
    transexamic acid 105–6
    uterine problems 96–101
metformin 126–7, 165–7, 178
Microgynon 61, 105, 115
Minoxidil 68
Minulet 115
Mirena device 106, 114, 144, 177
miscarriage 142–3
mood changes 61
multifollicular ovaries 22

nafarelin 97, 99
norethisterone 97, 103

oestradiol 11, 53, 74
oestrogen 6, 9, 10–11, 12, 50, 53, 54, 74,
    150
oestrone 11
osteoporosis 88, 175
ovarian cancer 176
ovarian cyst 133
ovarian dysfunction 5
ovaries 2–3, 13–15, 21–2, 39
ovulation 6, 122–7, 144, 148, 165–9

phytoestrogens 41, 45
Pill see contraceptive Pill
pituitary gland 8, 12, 38, 84–7
polycystic ovaries (PCO) 6, 16, 17, 174,
    180, 183–5
    and pain 22
    definition 1–4, 5
    diagnosis 19–30
polycystic ovary syndrome (PCOS) 4–6,
    16, 17, 174–5, 180–1, 185
    and cancer 177, 178, 179

and contraceptive Pill 36, 37, 118–19
and diet 39–42, 45, 148, 181, 184
and eating disorders 39, 40
and environment 39–42
and female foetus 39
and fertility 111–13, 122, 142–5
and genetic inheritance 32–4, 44
and heart disease 177
and insulin 148, 150, 164–5, 182
and menstrual problems 73–80
and Mirena device 106, 114
and ovulation 122–5, 126–7, 156–7,
   165–9
and sugar 148
and weight maintenance 42, 75, 76,
   77, 78, 148, 156–62, 181,
   184
causes 32–45
diagnosis 6, 19–30
insulin resistance (IR) 28, 39, 43,
   126, 128, 149–62, 172, 182
laparoscopic surgery 140–2
permanency of 44
thousand cases study 49–50, 76, 77,
   111, 113
twin studies 34–7, 40, 181
pregnancy outcomes, PCO and PCOS
   142–4
progesterone 6–7, 9, 11–12, 125
progesterone blood test 125
progestin 61, 99–100, 105, 115
prolactin levels 82–3
prostate cancer 48–9, 183
scalp hair loss 26, 46, 54, 68, 70
sex hormone binding globulin (SHBG)
   10, 16, 43, 52, 73, 74, 77, 150
sex hormones
   production 9–12
   regulation 12–15
Sheehan's syndrome 87
skin problems 4, 16, 46, 50–4
spironolactone 66, 183
sterilisation 120–1
stress and menstruation 81–2

sugar
   and insulin 158–9
   and PCOS 148, 157
Syndrome X 150, 177
Synacthen test 93–4

testosterone 9, 10, 12, 16, 28, 48, 49, 53,
   54–5, 74, 149, 164–5
tetracyclines 60
thyroid gland 29, 55, 83, 89–91
topical eflornithine 67–8
transexamic acid 26, 105–6
triglycerides 28, 119, 150, 162–4, 172
trimethoprim 60
Tri-Minulet 115
Trioden-ED 115
Triphasil 61
Triquilar 61
tumours 86–7
Turner's syndrome 88
twin studies 34–7, 40

ultrasound scanning 2, 5, 20–1, 29
uterine cancer 102, 114, 119, 176, 177,
   178, 179
uterine problems 96–101

vaginal ultrasound 20–1, 29

websites 201–5
weight loss
   and insulin resistance (IR) 170,
      172
   diets 157, 172–3
and glycaemic index (GI) 157, 158,
   159–62, 163
and ovulation 126–7, 148, 156–62
and PCOS 42, 75, 76, 77, 78, 148.
   156–62. 181, 184
see also body mass index (BMI)

Yasmin 61, 105, 115–16

zinc supplements 68–9